MW00861952

PEDORTHICS 101

For
Your
Foot Health

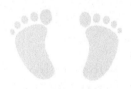

Root Cause of Foot Problems
How to Eliminate the Cause
Anklebone Alignment Test
Correct Walking

Inna Chon, Pedorthist

Pedorthics 101
For Your Foot Health.

Copyright © Inna Chon, 2017

All rights reserved. No part of this publication may be reproduced, distributed, or transmitted in any form or by any means, including photocopying, recording, or other electronic or mechanical methods, without the prior written permission of the publisher, except in the case of brief quotations embodied in critical reviews and certain other noncommercial uses permitted by copyright law.

Contact info: feetbalanceorthotics@gmail.com

Revised: October 2023
First Published in the United States of America in 2017
Publisher: Feet Balance Orthotics LLC

Library Congress Control Number: 2017912245
ISBN: 978-1-947142-01-5 (paperback black & white)
ISBN: 978-1-947142-02-2 (paperback full color)
ISBN: 978-1-947142-00-8 (eBook)

Cover and Interior Design by Inna Chon
Illustrations by Inna Chon

My Credentials

I am a certified pedorthist since 2005. I gained my pedorthic education from "The Foot and Ankle Institute of Temple University" in Philadelphia, Pennsylvania.

I majored in physical therapy at the Korea Medical College in South Korea. After I came to the United States, I was given an opportunity to become an animator. And later, mysteriously and thankfully, I received a call from the Disney Feature Animation Studio and worked there for 16 movies. While with Disney, I took evening courses for fashion design at the Fashion Institute of Design and Merchandising (FIDM) in Los Angeles, California. Interestingly, all three of these backgrounds have greatly contributed to my training, practice, and ongoing research in the pedorthic field.

My physical therapy background helps me to understand how to treat foot problems without medication or surgery.

As an animator, I know how to analyze movement with weight and ground reaction force, which the foot has to handle every day and cannot miss any subtle movement in order to draw out natural movements for the big screen. After understanding an object's structure and its mechanics, animators draw the movement of the object (usually with some exaggeration) in fractions of the movement up to twenty-four drawings per second, and they are scanned into a computer to ensure that the movement on the screen is smooth and natural. It takes well-trained eyes to catch any unnatural movement, especially, in slow motions, even half the thin mechanical pencil's lead thickness can cause wobbling in the movements. When that happens, the problematic drawings have to be located, and that subtle thickness has to be adjusted. With that skill and knowledge, I thoroughly analyzed the foot structure and its mechanics, especially, during the weight bearing stage (the stance phase) in the walking cycle, then I demonstrated that the orthotics are the essential devices for aligning anklebones, which is critical for the balance of our feet and the entire body alignment as well.

Finally, my fashion design background tells me that the orthotics should become a sought-after fashion item in the near future—just like eyeglasses.

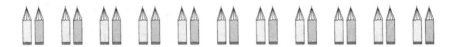

Table of Contents

CHAPTER 9

CHAPTER 10

CHAPTER 11

FALLEN TARSAL JOINT & ACHING FOOT ------------------------------- 125

CHAPTER 12

PROBLEMS ABOVE THE FOOT -- 138

CHAPTER 13

OVERALL BODY PERFORMANCES --- 150

Preface

Our body stands on the anklebones. Thus, it's important to "Align both Anklebones at the Same Height. "

But, both anklebones of most people are all tilted in different degrees and angles. This usually makes one leg shorter than the other and make people to limp. Limping means that our body is moving without the alignment.

When a body is moving without the alignment, the body cannot use its full strength and cannot use its full range of motion, and the body has to compensate all the time. Also, soon or later the weight-bearing joints will get damaged and cause pain.

If we don't align both anklebones at the same height first, all the treatments are done without the alignment, and all the healings are taking place without the alignment. So, nothing can be done properly.

So, for the overall body health and its ultimate functionality, we need to align both anklebones at the same height. Then our body finally can stand and move with alignment from the feet up. Then our body can use its full strength and its full range of motion without compensating.

And I found out how to the "Anklebone Alignment Test," which can tell if both anklebones are aligned at the same height or not. I do believe once our healthcare industry incorporates this "Anklebone Alignment Test" in the healthcare protocol, all the treatments for the structural and mechanical problems in our body will be done more efficiently with simpler procedure and less costs, and the overall body health will improve in a sensible way, since aligning both anklebones at the same height eliminates the root cause of the most structural and mechanical problems in our body.

We all have only one body and should make sure it moves with alignment. The alignment of every standing structure starts at the bottom. So, the alignment of our body starts at the bottom too, at the feet.

The definition of the word "foot" from the "www.dictionary.com" is as follows: the terminal part of the leg, below the ankle joint on which the body stands and moves, and such a part considered as the organ of locomotion. The Internet dictionary states simply as the "lower extremity of the leg below the ankle on which a person stands or walks."

The above statements indicate that the foot is the foundation of our body, but no one talks about how it is constructed with the "Tarsal Joint" that forms the arch. And when we make a step our entire body weight has to pass through this Tarsal Joint, and this Tarsal Joint has a tiny, 1-2mm of up-and-down range of motion.

So, if we don't support this tarsal joint with correct orthotics, this "Tarsal joint" falls from its tiny range of motion with each step and puts the entire foot bones out of alignment including the anklebone on which the leg bone stands. This, systematically, puts the entire body structure out of alignment.

However, most people do not realize this "Tarsal joint" in our foot has been falling little by little with each step since we were toddlers causing structural and mechanical problems throughout the body.

Our foot is constantly moving up and down with our moving body structure on it with about 98% of our entire body weight. This makes the small foot the moving foundation with a relatively tall moving structure on it. Doesn't its job sound pretty heavy? Still, most of us take them for granted and not giving them proper attention until our foot screams with pain or with some serious deformities.

The health of our foot is deeply related to our whole body's well-being; from the way we walk to our frowning faces from the foot-related discomforts. Yet, no one really talks about the matter at hand. I believe the Bible as the "Instruction from the Manufacturer of the Human Body Machine." So, I thought it would be unfair if this foot issue were not mentioned in the "Instruction," since it is so critical for our body machine's proper functionality. So, I searched the "Instruction" for the verses with the word, "Foot" that address this issue accordingly . . . And, yes..!

There it was! In the perfect place…!! Right after it tells us to "Strengthen our feeble arms and weak knees" in the Instruction of Hebrew chapter 12, verse12, the verse13 addresses the matter quite clearly in just ONE sentence . . !

"Make level paths for your feet, so that the lame may not be disabled, but rather be healed." (NIV)

Another translation reads:

"Make straight paths for your feet, so that what is lame may not be put out of joint but rather be healed." (ESV)

If I decipher this passage correctly, the unleveled path for the feet makes people limp (the lame) and eventually may make them disabled or put them out of joint. To be healed from disabling or joint problems, we need to make level paths or straight paths "For our Feet."

Many scientific facts are found in the "Instruction." And this sentence is another scientific fact, in this case, "How to take care of our joints."

Once we understand the foot structure with the "Tarsal Joint" that forms the arch, the "leveled" or "straight" paths referenced in these verses should not be interpreted literally as leveled or straight grounds. Because on those leveled or straight grounds, the "Tarsal Joint" definitely falls misaligning the entire foot bones including the anklebone on which our body stands. So, if we read between the lines, the proper level paths or straight paths for the feet should be the paths that level or align the foot bones.

Also, this passage from the "Instruction" definitely implies that the limping (the human body machine moving without the alignment) is related to the feet, which is a common sense since the foot is the foundation of our body. But most of us are oblivious to the fact that the foot is engineered with the "Tarsal Joint" that needs support to keep the entire foot bones and our body structure in alignment. A body with alignment, we cannot limp (although we can pretend to be limping). Without the alignment . . .? We cannot NOT limp.

> "Most of the fundamental ideas of science are essentially simple, and may, as a rule, be expressed in a language comprehensible to everyone." (Albert Einstein)

By applying the basic laws of physics, how to keep the "Tarsal Joint" from falling and the method of the "Anklebone Alignment Test" or even the "Hip bone Alignment Test" and how to stand and walk correctly become essentially simple. So, as a rule, it may be expressed in a language that is comprehensible to everyone.

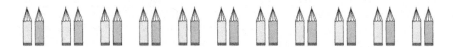

Chapter 1

In the Beginning

The Foot & Soft Ground

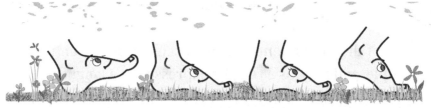

The human foot is created with an arch at the bottom that meant to be supported and supposed to walk on soft soil with barefoot. In the beginning, mist would come up from the earth and watered the whole face of the ground (Gen 2:6).

This would mean the soil was able to keep itself soft all the time even after the foot stepped on it. Then this ever-soft soil would fill and support the arch area all the time and kept the tarsal joint from falling. It is like planting the foot into the soil.

Interestingly, the word "plantar" refers to the bottom of the foot. This word came from the word "plant,' which means to place into the soil. So, when walking on the soft soil, the foot bottom and a little bit of all around the foot at the bottom were planted into the soil like a root, like the above drawing; then the foot was able to carry our body weight while keeping the tarsal joint from falling.

I think this was the condition of the soil in the Garden before God cursed the ground. Because, after God cursed the ground (Genesis 3:17), Adam was to till the ground (Genesis 3:23). The purpose of tilling is to soften the ground, isn't it?

The condition of the soil before and after the curse must be different.

Destroyer of the Foot

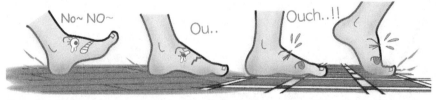

Gradually the ground became harder, and the industrialization changed the ground with the flat and hard concrete—no means of filling and supporting the arch. The flat and hard grounds should be considered as destroyers of the foot. Because, on these grounds, the tarsal joint definitely falls and puts the entire foot structure and the body structure out of alignment. The carpets and cushy floors are little better only for the fatty tissues at the bottom of the heel and the ball of the foot, but they cannot keep the tarsal joint from falling. The flatter and harder the floor, the harder it is on the foot. Walking on the flat and hard surfaces will damage our foot along with our major weight-bearing joints much faster than on the soft ground.

As no one will walk with barefoot on the streets covered with broken glasses in fear of damaging the skin, we should not walk on the flat surfaces without the correct orthotics in fear of damaging the tarsal joint. The flat and hard surfaces are for man-made subjects, such as automobiles, machines, and furniture but not for the human foot with the arch at the bottom. If the human body keeps walking on the flat surfaces, one day, our body will also become a machine with iron rods and screws—still without the alignment.

☆ Think about This

We wouldn't want to use a flat-bottomed computer on a rounded surface as it fluctuates and shakes all the time; this will damage the computer's hardware and even can mess up the software down the road. A flat-bottomed object should be placed on flat surface for balance and stability.

Likewise, our foot with an arch at the bottom should not walk on flat surfaces, because it will block the circulation at the heel and ball of the foot areas, and the tarsal joint that forms the arch will be fluctuating and shaking as it falls; this will stress our body physically (hardware) and mentally (software). Yet, we are doing this to our own "body machine," which cannot be replaced.

If our foot were created without the arch at the bottom, we could only walk like ducks, and never be able to run and jump in all kinds of activities; because without the arch, our foot and all the major joints cannot handle the impact or ground reaction force that comes from running or jumping. That is why being flat-footed is an issue if trying to join the military. Also, even with the orthotics, it is good to walk on the soft ground as it can absorb more of the ground reaction force from under the foot. This reduces the impact on the foot and the major weight-bearing joints above the foot.

Perhaps you already have a lot of knowledge about the foot and how to care for foot problems. But, here and now, if you can set aside everything you know and start with a blank slate and an open mind with a foot bone structure in front of you; you can discover something new and very true.

Now, let's start analyzing foot structure.

Chapter 2

Foot Structure with Tarsal Joint

In This Chapter
- Bones & Joints
- Muscles, Tendons, & Ligaments
    - Intrinsic Muscles & Ligaments
    - Extrinsic Tendons
  - Muscle Characteristics
  - Interesting Facts about the Tarsal Joint

Bones & Joints

There are 28 bones per foot (so 56 bones for both feet).

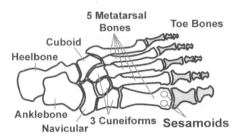

Many sources say that there are 26 bones per foot not counting the 2 sesamoid bones right under the 1st metatarsal head. Their function is to reduce the impact on the 1st metatarsal head area while protecting its joint when standing and walking.

The current medical study divides the foot into three parts: hindfoot, midfoot, and forefoot . . . like below.

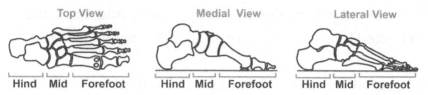

But it is kind of confusing to understand since it mixes the arch and the toes together. It would be much easier to understand if we divide the foot into two parts: the arch and the toes—as they appear to be in the structure . . . like below.

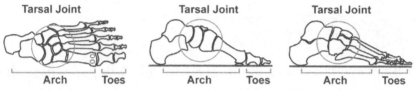

The arch is constructed with the "Tarsal Joint" and 2 small sesamoids. This tarsal joint is the most complicated joint in our body not many people know about, and the toes are in front of the arch. They share the same number of bones; 14 bones make up the arch, and 14 bones make up the 5 toes—easy to remember. The heel and the ball of the foot are both end parts of the arch that touch the ground.

Let's move on with the arch and the toe divisions . . .

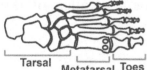

The toes are like short version of fingers, and we can tell there are joints since we can wiggle them around. Each toe is made of 2 bones (big toe), or 3 bones (4 small toes) of rather small and similar shapes. So, together, 14 toe bones make 14 joints. And each toe is connected to each head of the 5 metatarsal bones.

How about the arch? The arch is formed by the tarsal joint on top of the foot. This tarsal joint involves 12 foot bones: 7 tarsal bones, 5 metatarsal bones. The 7 tarsal bones are very different in shapes and sizes, while 5 metatarsal bones are similar in shape and size.

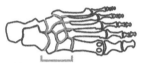

Tarsal/Arch Joint
Compared to the 5 wiggly toes, the outside look of the arch is like . . . a lump . . . without any joint. But those 12 foot bones with different shapes and sizes are arranged like a 3D puzzle making about 20 small joints on top of the arch (hard to count due to its complexity; so instead of giving each joint a name, we just call the entire group of these small joints the "Tarsal Joint"). This puzzle-like connection leaves the tarsal joint with a very limited range of motion, only about 1-2mm of up and down motion that works as a shock absorber. We can move this Tarsal Joint by flexing the toes up and down. However, due to its very tiny range of motion, we cannot see much of the movement.

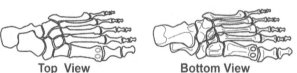

Top View   **Bottom View**   The view from the top and bottom of the tarsal joint look very different;

while the top-view remains smooth (we can feel it because there is only a thin layer of muscle partially covering the top of the arch area), the bottom-view has a very jagged appearance due to the 5 small tarsal bones having very irregular wedge shapes at the bottom. However, it's impossible to feel those jagged joints due to the thick plantar ligaments and muscles right under the Tarsal Joint.

(It is interesting that the foot bones that carry the entire body weight are the smallest among the other weight-bearing bones. I think this makes the foot bones to have less chance to be broken, though the joints can be sprained.)

Muscles, Tendons & Ligaments

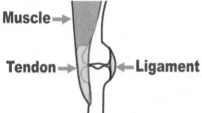

Muscles have the ability to contract and relax to make the joints move. The tendons connect muscles to bones, the ligaments connect bones to bones (tendon and ligament do not have much flexibility). There are two kinds of foot muscles: intrinsic muscles and extrinsic muscles.

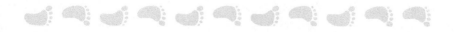

14

Intrinsic Muscles & Ligaments

The foot intrinsic muscles and ligaments are the ones that connect the 28 foot bones together and hold the shape of the foot. They are mostly short in length, but the ligaments that connect the tarsal joint can be considered the strongest ligaments in our body. There are not many intrinsic muscles, but around 100 ligaments connecting those rather small 28 foot bones. And while just one layer of thin short ligaments connects the top of the tarsal joint, there are many layers of short, medium, and long plantar ligaments fill right under the tarsal joint.

Right under the many layers of the plantar ligaments is filled with 4 layers of thick plantar muscles. (We can call this group of muscles the "arch muscles" since the muscles fill the arch area only.) These plantar muscles work as a built-in cushion. And there are thick fatty tissues right under the heel bone and the heads of the metatarsal bones (the ball of the foot area) working as the pad to protect these bones from about 25% of our body weight.

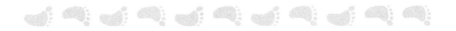

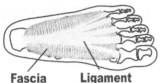

Fascia   **Ligament**   Right under the plantar muscles is the tight plantar fascia ligament (the longest ligament of the foot). This plantar fascia ligament runs from the front part of the heel bone and branches out into 5 narrow ligaments, and each attach to each head of the metatarsal bones. But the one that attached to the first metatarsal head is the thickest and tightest. We can feel this tight ligament by pressing over the medial arch area with fingers while lifting the toes all up.

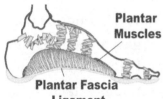

Plantar Muscles

Plantar Fascia Ligament   From all around this ligament spread out sheets of fascia (connective tissues) wrapping and binding the ligament and the plantar muscles tightly to the bottom of the tarsal joint and shape the arch at the bottom. This arch is the part needs the support from the correct orthotics to keep the tarsal joint falling while carrying the 75% of the body weight.

Imagine what will happen when the entire body weight passing through the unsupported tarsal joint. This puts the entire body weight on the heel and the ball of the foot area only, and the tarsal joint would surely fall . . . Isn't it scary? Even though the foot is made with just one piece of bone, the arch is better be supported for even weight distribution for a good circulation.

Extrinsic Tendons

Extrinsic tendons are the tendons of the leg muscles, and they are the ones that move the foot. As the leg muscles go down toward the foot, they all become tendons and pass the ankle joint and attach to diffident foot bones. There are 12 leg muscles, but only 11 tendons pass the ankle joint because 2 leg muscles (gastrocnemius and soleus) join into the Achilles tendon and attach to the back of the heel bone. Most of the extrinsic tendons attach to the foot bones that make up the tarsal joint, and a few tendons attach to the toe bones to move the toes.

Muscle Characteristics

The flexibility of muscles and ligaments and their volumes are hereditary factors. Some people are born with tight ligaments/muscles that do not stretch easily, while others are born with flexible ligaments/muscles that stretch easily. Also, some people are born with thick, voluminous muscles (these people may also have thick voluminous plantar muscles, which makes their arches look low), while some are born with thin, lanky muscles (these people may also have thin plantar muscles, which makes their arches look high).

It seems that if your ancestors were originally from cold weather regions, such as northern Europe, most likely you may have inherited the tight muscles, and if your ancestors were from warm weather regions, such as Africa or South America, most likely you may have inherited the flexible muscles. No wonder the African American basketball players can maneuver their body faster and more smoothly through the players than the northern Europeans.

Also, it seems that when the body is moving without the alignment due to the fallen tarsal joint, people with tight muscles tend to be able to keep the slim body shapes, while people with soft and flexible muscles tend to easily develop obesity (it would be an interesting subject for further research).

Interesting Facts about the Tarsal Joint

First of all, we should call the tarsal joint as the "Major weight-bearing joint", and all other weight-bearing joints that stand on the tarsal joint should be called as the "Secondary weight-bearing joints." Because the tarsal joint is the one that carries the most body weight.

Structure-wise, this tarsal joint is totally opposite of the other weight-bearing joints.

First of all, it is arranged in a side-by-side manner to form the arch like a 3D puzzle, while the other weight-bearing joints are standing on top of each other. So, the tarsal joint needs the correct support—the correct orthotics—from under to keep it from falling and so to keep it in alignment.

And most foot muscles are around the tarsal joint, mostly at the bottom of the tarsal joint, while the other weight-bearing joints do not have muscles around the joints, rather they are around the shaft of the bones.

Even though the tarsal joint carries the most body weight than the other weight-bearing joints, there is no weight between those small joints in the tarsal joint, while most weight-bearing joints get the weight between the joints.

When the tarsal joint goes out of alignment, those small joint rather spread out (unless the shoes are too tight), so even though the fallen tarsal joint is the root cause of the pain at the bottom of the foot (such as the heel, arch, ball of the foot, and the toe areas) and in the major joints, the tarsal joint itself on top of the foot do not have pain.

That is why people overlook the root cause of the joint pain, the fallen tarsal joint on top of the foot. So, all the treatments are done without eliminating the root cause.

Interesting . . .

Chapter 3

Purpose of Alignment

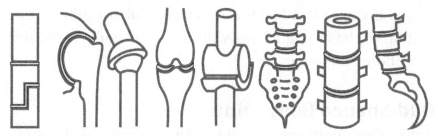

Every machine needs proper alignment. It's so crucial for a machine to function well and last long. We all know this fact. Then what does alignment essentially provide for the machine to run smoothly or function well and last long? Most people have a hard time answering this question, just saying, "Because it is . . . aligned . . ," or "It's aligned, that is why . . ." But the question is to explain what the 'alignment provides' for the machine to run smoothly and last long.

Even Weight Distribution

The answer is "Even Weight Distribution." Alignment = Even Weight Distribution = Minimal Deterioration = Optimal Functionality. Every object on earth is subject to gravity, and every joint in a machine deteriorates from weight or pressure even with the proper alignment. Without the alignment, joints get a greater and faster deterioration—due to uneven weight distribution. Especially, the area that deals with a heavy weight or pressure, the alignment has to be very precise. For example, auto mechanics know how the weight from a small piece of lead on a wheel affects the alignment of the entire automobile. Like a wheel, our small foot carries tremendous weight. therefore, it needs the precise alignment as well. So, when we make orthotics, even less than a half millimeter height mistake can affect the even weight distribution at the bottom of the foot, and this will make our body to fail the Anklebone Alignment test.

Odd-Shaped Body Joints

Our body's joints are irregularly shaped with all different ranges of motion. This makes it hard to tell if any angle of a given joint is within its normal range of motion, or from out of alignment. However, we can differentiate between the two with the "strength test." If the angle of a joint is within its range of motion, the body should be able to utilize its full strength. But even a slightest angle of the joint is from out of alignment, the body cannot utilize its full strength.

Ironically, we, human beings, who know every machine should be aligned before being put into operation, do not apply that concept to our own body machine, and do not know how to align our body exactly.

Also, the body alignment has to be checked in a standing posture starting from the feet up, not from somewhere in the middle or in a lying down posture. If you ask someone, "What part of our body controls the alignment of the entire body?" most likely, the answer will be "the spine."

But the spine is standing on the hip bones. And most hip bones are in a tilted position (due to the fallen tarsal joint). That is why most spine stands without the alignment. However, if the spine is the one that can align the entire body structure, can the spine somehow stand straight on its own on the tilted hip bones and pull the hip bones in alignment? Or can the spine somehow align both anklebones way at the bottom at the same height? Very confusing to even think about, because it is totally against the basic theory of the law of physics. In order to align the spine, needless to say, the hip bones have to be aligned first. In order to align the hip bones, the two legs have to stand with the same length (or height). In order for two legs to stand with the same length, both anklebones have to be aligned at the same height from the ground.

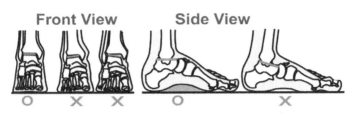

Front View   **Side View**

Once we observe the foot structure and see how the anklebone is situated, we will all agree that without the correct orthotics, the anklebones cannot be aligned, so our entire body structure also.

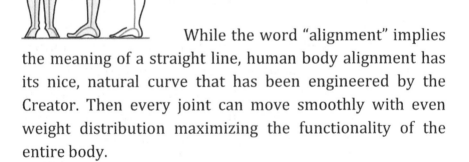

While the word "alignment" implies the meaning of a straight line, human body alignment has its nice, natural curve that has been engineered by the Creator. Then every joint can move smoothly with even weight distribution maximizing the functionality of the entire body.

From the above side-view illustrations, notice that the optimal head position is to look up to heaven at a 45-degree angle. This position divides the head weight equally over the neck bone freeing all the neck muscles from stress (I guess the Creator wants us to look up to Him; so whenever possible, look up and talk.)

In any posture, every arched area on the ground should be supported accordingly for even weight distribution throughout the body surface at the bottom. This helps the blood circulation while keeping our body's natural curves.

When a person lies down on their back, several arched areas appear at the bottom that would need the support for even weight distribution: the arches under the back of the neck, lower back, back of the knees, and back of the ankles. This will also help long-term bedridden people to prevent bedsores on shoulders, hips, and the back of the heels.

Though, these supports do not have to be accurate for even weight distribution since the weight the supports carrying is not really heavy.

(Tips for the supports: Under the back of the neck, use a small half-tube- pillow to make the head to tilt backwards and rest the back of the head comfortably on the bed. Under the lower back, choose a correct thickness of rectangular shape pillow long enough to roll over on it sideways. This also helps the digestive system with more space by raising the tummy-side up. Under the back of the knees, use a small pillow just enough to give a little support. Lastly, under the back of the ankles, use a pillow thick enough to lift the heels off the bed. This will free the heels from any weight bearing, so the blood can circulate nicely around the heel.)

When lying down on the sideways, the under the side of the neck and head and the side of the waist area need the comfortable support.

But beware, a pillow under the non-arched area will ruin the body's natural curve; for example, a pillow under the back of the head without the enough support beneath the neck area can mass up the neck's natural curve and end up with a straight neck.

Now, when we are standing, only two arches, one on each foot, need the support with the orthotics. This support for the arch has to be very precise to align the anklebones to spread the entire body weight evenly throughout the bottom of the foot. The arch part alone should carry about 75% of the body weight and 25% of it goes to the heel and the ball of the foot areas.

Heavily Abused Foot

When we stand and walk, the entire body weight goes to the bottom of the foot. However, people don't think about how much weight our foot have to handle each day.

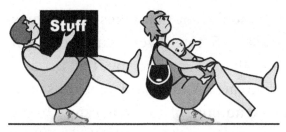

Let's find out how much weight each foot has to handle every day. For an easy calculation, let's use a person weighs only 100 pounds, which is a fairly lightweight for a body weight in general. However, when we try to lift it, 100 pounds is a lot of weight (try to lift it to get the feel of it). Imagine that much, or more, weight falls on one foot each step we make. Without the correct orthotics, all that weight only goes to the heel and the ball of the foot areas, but not the arch area.

On average, a person takes 5,000 to 10,000 steps a day. Let's choose a person who walks 5,000 steps a day (who is not really active). This means one foot carries 100 pounds with every step.

A 100 pound person who walks 5,000 steps:

Number of steps per foot: 5,000 ÷ 2 = 2,500 steps.
Multiply by the person's weight: 2,500 × 100 = 250,000 lbs.

Wow, that's too big of a number to imagine in pound. Let's convert that into tons.

1 ton is about 2000 lbs.: 250,000 ÷ 2000 = 125 tons.

Wow . . . a 100 pound person's foot that takes 2,500 steps has to deal with at least 125 tons every day, not even considering the impact that is caused by the ground reaction force, or stuffs we carry. You can calculate this with your own body weight and number of your daily steps to get an idea. For monthly or yearly weight, multiply by 30 or 365, and for total weight to the present day, multiply yearly weight by your age.

In order to minimize the damage caused by the weight, the even weight distribution is necessary on the surface where the weight falls. Also, maximizing the weight-bearing surface is the wise thing.

Chapter 4

Fallen Tarsal Joint

In This Chapter
- The Tarsal Joint Should Not Fall
- Orthotics & Pedorthics

Not many people heard of the word, "Tarsal Joint.," especially, the "Fallen Tarsal Joint." There are many Internet sites about the "fallen arch." Though, the fallen arch causes many serious symptoms, there is no explanation as to how this "fallen arch" came into existence in the first place, how to prevent it from happening, or how to correct it. Although, the "fallen arch" is the outside look of the "Fallen Tarsal Joint."

These days, people of all age suffer from major joint and muscle pain, foot deformities, aching feet, poor posture, scoliosis, and other complicated structural and mechanical problems. These are often thought of as hereditary, or natural phenomena as our body ages, or as the unknown cause (idiopathy). Yes, aging is one of the factors that cause problems, but the root cause of the above problems is resting on the "Fallen Tarsal Joint" on top of the foot that no one talk about.

The Tarsal Joint Should Not Fall

Tarsal/Arch Joint

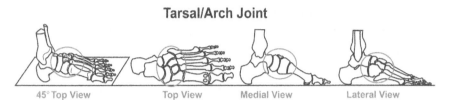

45° Top View   Top View   Medial View   Lateral View

The group of tiny joints on top of the foot is the "Tarsal Joint." First thing we should notice is that when we stand, while all the weight-bearing bones above the foot are stacked on top of each other on the anklebone (Talus), all of the foot bones are arranged in a side-by-side manner except the anklebone sits askew on the heel bone and those 2 sesamoids under the 1st metatarsal head.

The structure of the foot is totally opposite of the other weight-bearing joints above the foot that are stacked on top of each other on the anklebone. So, this Tarsal Joint's side-by-side arrangement do not put the body weight between the small joints. Rather, when the Tarsal Joint falls and goes out of alignment, the space between those small joints in the Tarsal Joint spread out making the foot wider and longer, whereas the other weight-bearing joints on top of the foot are squeezed by the weight while being out of alignment (the reason our foot gets bigger and bigger, and our height get shorter and shorter). So, there rarely a pain in the Tarsal Joint while the other weight bearing joints screaming with pain. We know the joint pain usually triggers by weight bearing while being out of alignment. This "No Pain" is the reason people do not pay attention to the Tarsal Joint; even though most people have the "Fallen Tarsal Joint."—No wonder why we are dealing with many cause-unknown (idiopathic) symptoms.

This puzzle-like Tarsal Joint has a very tiny, about 1-2mm of up and down range of motion that works as a shock absorber. When we make a step, our entire body weight has to pass through this Tarsal Joint. When there is no correct orthotics under the tarsal joint, these tiny side-by-side joints fall and misalign the entire foot bones including the anklebone on which the leg bone stands. This is the "Fallen Tarsal Joint" that is known as the "fallen arch." Since the "Fallen Tarsal Joint" tilts the anklebone, the entire major joints that stand on the anklebone systematically go out of alignment at the same time; this causes structural and mechanical problems throughout our body. (Shouldn't we teach this fact from elementary schools .. ?)

This Tarsal Joint begins to fall when toddlers start to stand and walk on the flat surfaces if not using the correct orthotics under the arch, and it keeps falling every step we make as long as we live, or until complete collapse. This fallen tarsal joint makes our body moving without the alignment from the feet up until we use the correct orthotics that aligning both anklebones at the same height.

Orthotics & Pedorthics

Let's go over a little bit of the history of the orthotics and pedorthics.

There are shreds of evidence that the ancient people, like 2,000 years ago, used some soft materials—like wool or leather—to support their arches to ease the foot pain. However, the modern orthotics have been around for over 100 years in the United States. Still, some people have never heard of the word, "Orthotics."

The definition of the word "Pedorthics" from the website "opcareers.org" reads as follow: "The science and practice of evaluating, fabricating, delivery of footwear and foot orthoses to prevent or improve painful or disabling conditions of the foot and ankle caused by disease, congenital defects, overuse, or injury." And it was followed by "The word 'Pedorthics' first appeared in medical dictionaries in 1980, although the field itself began to emerge in the late 1950's after World War II, and an outbreak of polio created a need to deal with foot trauma and deformities." Even though there are a lot of pedorthic information on the Internet, the word "Pedorthics" is not displayed in every dictionary yet.

So, not many people heard of the words "pedorthics" or "pedorthist," though the Pedorthic Footcare Association (PFA) has been around since 1958. The meaning of the word "ped-" is the "foot" and "-orthist" is the "one who aligns." Thus, the pedorthist's job should be providing the correct orthotics that aligning the foot bones—especially, **Both Anklebones at the Same Height**. And this should be the first agenda in pedorthic protocol, and then pedorthist should teach people how to walk correctly through the medial arch, understanding the foot anatomy in connection with the weight bearing.

Most people confuse pedorthist with podiatrist. It is like confusing optometrist with ophthalmologist. We all know that the ophthalmologist is the one who prescribes drugs and performs surgery, whereas the optometrist is the one who provides eyeglasses for a good vision, and they do the vision test with the lenses first and then after they put the lenses into the eyeglass frame to check if the frame is leveled or not. Similarly, the podiatrist is the one who prescribes drugs and performs surgery, whereas the pedorthist is the one who provides orthotics that align both anklebones at the same height for the genuine foot balance and comfort.

However, most orthotics and shoes are being dispensed merely to alleviate the pressure at the bottom of the foot for a "temporary comfort." To provide the "lasting comfort" is to spread the body weight evenly throughout the bottom of the foot including the arch area. This even weight distribution also helps the blood circulation at the bottom of the foot, thus, helps the healing process of whatever the problems at the bottom of the foot. This, also, helps the circulation of the entire body system too, since our body is all connected to each other.

To spread the body weight evenly at the bottom of foot, both anklebones should be aligned at the same height. So, the pedorthists should do the "Anklebone Alignment Test" when dispensing the orthotics to make sure the orthotics are aligning people's both anklebones at the same height. So, when people are getting the orthotics from pedorthists, they are aligning their both anklebones at the same height.

The orthotics that aligning both anklebones at the same height also aligns our entire body structure that stand on the anklebones, so, provides our entire body with balance and comfort. Thus, providing the correct orthotics is imperative and vital for the overall human body health.

So, the orthotics' main function should be realigning the "Fallen Tarsal Joint" to the point of aligning both anklebones at the same height. This calls for the "Anklebone Alignment Test," or simply the "AA test," which I found out how to do and coined the name. (It will be discussed in detail in chapter 9). This "Anklebone Alignment Test" is the missing piece in the pedorthic practice, so it should be incorporated in the pedorthic practice soon as possible.

This "Anklebone Alignment Test" is like the "vision test" in optometric practice. So, the "Anklebone Alignment Test" should be done with the orthotics first and after putting the orthotics into the shoes to check if the shoe bottoms are leveled or not. And orthotics are very accurate devices that demands less than 1/2-millimeter accuracy, and the pedorthist should explain how to walk correctly, which will be discussed in chapter 6.

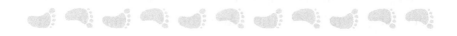

Since most orthotics are still dispensed without the "Anklebone Alignment Test," most orthotics do not exactly align people's both anklebones at the same height. So, people are not getting full benefits of the orthotics, and some are experiencing more problems with the orthotics than before. Because some ill-fitted orthotics can misalign the wearer's anklebones worse than before. Consequently, a very small percentage of people are using orthotics even though it is the essential device not just for our feet but also for our overall body health, as mentioned before.

Furthermore, some people think the orthotics as some kind of crutches or braces. But remember, the support was there in the beginning with the soft soil. But now it's gone, and we are walking on the man-made flat floors. So, we need to use man-made orthotics to keep the tarsal joint from falling and keep the anklebones in alignment. Then finally, our body can stand and walk with alignment from the feet up, so can walk without limping.

The orthotics can be made with any methods and any materials. However, it would be more functional if they can go into many different types of shoes. And the "Anklebone Alignment Test" will enlighten people as to the importance of aligning the anklebones and bring the pedorthic practice to the forefront of healthcare practice. (Who doesn't need to align their anklebones?)

While analyzing the foot structure and its mechanics, I found that the current analysis of the foot is kind of complicated for the general public to understand and not quite relevant to the pedorthic practice. It can be analyzed and explained much simpler for easier understanding using the simple law of physics and, also, relevant to the pedorthic practice.

We all know the foundation of every object that stands on the ground has to be aligned. If not, the entire structure cannot be aligned (we don't need to go to school to know this). Without the alignment, the object cannot function properly. Similarly, without aligning the anklebones, our body cannot function properly, nor can last as long as it should, just like any man-made machine.

Before we go any further, it would be good to think about the purpose of alignment.

Chapter 5

The Arch

Where is the Arch

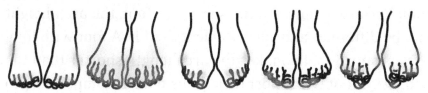

When we look at the foot, what do we see first? Yes, most likely 5 wiggly toes, possibly with brightly colored toenails. The arch . . .? Where is it? From where to where?

Even though it takes up most of the foot (technically, except for those 5 toes, the entire foot is the arch), it doesn't catch our eyes.

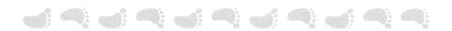

We can draw the arch line from the bottom of the heel bone and go up toward the bottom of the anklebone, and, from there, go down through the tarsal joint toward the ball of the foot. So the highest part of the arch is right under the anklebone on which the leg bone stands.

The height of the arch is hereditary, just like the height of our body. Some people are born with high arch, some with low arch. No one is born without the arch. We can see the arch in every newborn baby's foot. Flat foot happens when the tarsal joint collapses completely when standing on the flat floor. So, it should be called as "A foot with complete fallen tarsal joint." Doesn't it sound alarming?

Also, the size of the arch is not pertinent to the size of the foot. Because even with the same size foot, the arch height can be different, and, also, the length of it. A foot with long toes proportionally makes the arch length shorter than the same size foot with short toes. (This makes it impossible to integrate the orthotics into shoes without customizing to each individual.)

By observing all the joints in our body, we can see that this tarsal joint is the most complicated joint in our body; though, its outside appearance is simple.

Dividing the Arch

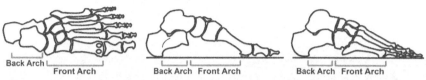

Back Arch ⌊_____⌋
   ⌊__⌋ ⌊__⌋
Front Arch   Back Arch Front Arch   Back Arch Front Arch

The arch can be divided by 2 parts: the "back arch" and the "front arch." The back arch consists of only 2 bones, (the heel bone and the anklebone). It is from the front of the heel bone at the bottom to the front of the anklebone. The front arch consists of 12 bones (including 2 sesamoids); it is from the front of the anklebone to the behind the ball of the foot. In this front arch, the tarsal joint is located. Structure-wise, the back arch is higher than the front arch, and when the front arch falls the back arch gives in.

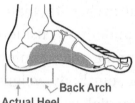

Back Arch

Actual Heel   The heel bone is the biggest foot bone with its back half touching the ground and the front half suspending in the air. So, the actual heel is the back half of the heel bone that touches the ground. But, due to the thick muscles filling in the back arch area, the back arch area appears to be part of the heel, but it is not.

The anklebone is the second-biggest foot bone sitting askew on the front part of the heel bone where it is suspended in the air. On top of this anklebone stands the leg bone. So, the body weight falls on the back arch.

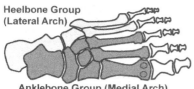

Heelbone Group (Lateral Arch)

Anklebone Group (Medial Arch)   Also, the arch can be divided by along the sideways: the high medial arch and the low lateral arch.

The high medial arch is formed by the group of bones attached to the front of the anklebone. We can call this group as the "anklebone group," which consist of 8 bones: the anklebone, navicular, 3 cuneiforms, and 3 (first, second, & third) metatarsal bones. This medial arch has much better shock absorber system than the lateral arch with many joints and much thicker plantar muscles under it to cushion tremendous weight and impact from running and jumping with whatever we carry—all day long. So, our body weight should fall straight down onto this high medial arch.

The low lateral arch is formed by the group of bones attached to the front of the heel bone. So, we can call this group as the "heel bone group," which consist of 4 bones: the heel bone, cuboid, and 2 metatarsal (fourth & fifth) bones. This lateral arch has few joints with thin plantar muscle under it to handle the residual body weight that passed down from the medial arch. Remember, even with the correct orthotics, the lateral arch is not designed to handle even just our body weight all day.

With the correct orthotics, our body weight should fall straight down onto the anklebone and pass through the center of the medial arch toward the second toe. This makes the foot to carry the entire body weight much more comfortably than walking with the body weight veering sideways and pass through the lateral arch.

Looking at the foot from behind, we can see the heel bone, anklebone, and the leg bone are all stacked off-centered toward the middle. This arrangement makes the body weight fall to where there is no structural support underneath. It is kind of scary to think about the entire body weight falling on that empty area. But the Creator filled that empty area with thick muscles as a built-in cushion. If that empty area were filled with a bone, it would crack in no time from the impact of the weight, and, that impact would shoot back up to all the (secondary) weight-bearing joints above the foot and add more stress to those joints.

When we stand with two feet right next to each other, the imaginary skeletal arch (transverse arch) is formed with the body weight falling on the middle top of it. This arrangement makes the arch less likely to fall laterally; thus, the legs would less likely bend outward where there is nothing to lean against; rather, if it ever falls, it will fall inward to where the two legs can lean against each other— Amazing design .. !

Linear Arches

Now, let's look at the bottom of the foot with the toes all up.

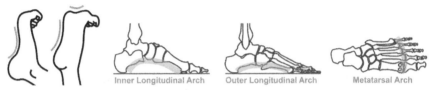

Inner Longitudinal Arch   Outer Longitudinal Arch   Metatarsal Arch

Then we can see the 3 linear arches: high medial arch (=Inner longitudinal arch), low lateral arch (=outer longitudinal arch), and the lowest metatarsal arch (= ball of the foot arch).

The medial arch runs along the medial side of the foot (big toe side). The lateral arch runs along the lateral side of the foot (pinky toe side), and the metatarsal arch runs across the ball of the foot.

As mentioned earlier, the arch part alone is the foundation of our body, as the whole body stands on the arch. The toes are in front of the arch for smooth transfer of the weight from the ball of the foot to the other foot while walking.

With all the above analyses, we can come up with 3 functions of the arch.

Functions of the Arch

As the foundation of our body, the arch has 3 functions.

1. Weight-bearing: The arch shape is the best-known structure for efficient weight bearing. And the weight should be evenly spread out throughout the arch area.

2. Shock absorber: The tarsal joint's tiny range of motion (about 1-2 mm) with the thick muscles under the arch absorbs the shock that occurs with every step.

3. Alignment of the major joints: The tarsal joint is responsible for the alignment of the entire body structure.

For the arch to perform the above 3 functions accordingly, we need to provide the correct orthotics that aligning both anklebones at the same height. It's like we need fill our stomach with health food for the stomach to do its job.

The bottom of the foot (though a very small area) is engineered to handle tremendous weight.

That is why a weightlifter lifts 1,000 lbs. even without the correct orthotics; so, just using the heel and the ball of the foot. Amazingly, our body is very precisely engineered, but it can tolerate quite a bit of abuse.

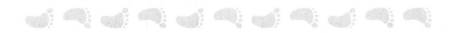 Because of this amazingly engineered foot bottom, people do not feel much weight at the bottom of the foot. (Curious? Put a finger under someone else's heel. This will hurt but instantly let you know.) It even jumps with a body carrying all kinds of stuffs.

Even with the correct orthotics, a 100 pound body generates a lot of pressure between the orthotics and the entire bottom of the foot. That is why even a grain of sand or a small lint from a sock inside of the shoes becomes bothersome and has to be removed. Because of this tightness, even one business card (less than a 1/2 mm thickness) between orthotics and the foot affects the even weight distribution at the bottom of the foot. Surprisingly, this breaks the balance, so the body will fail the Anklebone Alignment Test. It is like a slight invisible dent on an eyeglass lens, which distorts the vision. So, if we don't use the correct orthotics, we are torturing the foot to have deformities and pain.

To provide the balance and comfort for the foot, the body weight has to be evenly distributed throughout the bottom of the foot. Without the correct orthotics that aligning both anklebones at the same height, the even weight distribution at the bottom of the foot is not possible.

Functions of the foot

The foot has 2 functions: weight-bearing and walking.

The weight-bearing function is the arch part, and walking part is done by the joints at the ankle and the ball of the foot area. For the foot to perform these 2 functions properly, the foot joints should be in alignment. So, the correct orthotics are necessary to keep the tarsal joint in the arch area in alignment and the joints at ankle and the ball of the foot in alignment.

Unassertive Arch

Though this arch has very important roles for our overall body health, it's not getting its due attention. Why .. ? From the start, this humble arch is located at the very unassertive place—at the bottom ... with an unassertive appearance ... like a lump of flesh.

But, usually, hiding in the assertive shoes. Even with a bare foot, the attention all goes to those small assertive toes. Are they the women's toes? Then the arch cannot beat those assertively colored toenails. Even though the tarsal joint is completely fallen, the shape of a lump of flesh doesn't change much, while the heel and ball of the foot areas become assertive with calluses or pain, and toes are screaming with curls and twist. Also, our body structure that stands on the fallen tarsal joint becomes assertive with bad posture and joint pain, the fallen tarsal joint, most cases, still remains in silence.

The main reason for this would be the body weight falls on those clustered side-be-side 3D puzzle like joints. So there is no weight falls between the joints. And when the tarsal joint fall, the space between the joints rather spread apart over-stretching the ligaments—totally opposite from the other weight-bearing joints that stand on top of each other, as mentioned earlier.

Also, if there could be some stress in the tarsal joint, each of those 20 small joints only gets 1/20 of the total stress. And those small joints with 3D puzzle-like arrangement can compensate to many different directions and angles. So, if the pain is about to happen, the brain can shift the body weight to slightly different directions to alleviate the pain. And there are two feet to share the stress. So, the pain is unlikely to happen in the arch area.

But, from the ankle to knee to hip, which together make the leg, there is only one joint on top of each other to deal with the stress, and there are two legs, so they can alternate and share the stress.

Above the hip stands only one spine to deal with the stress with no other spine to share the stress. That is why most pain starts in the back, hips, knees, or the ankles . . . not in the arch, even though those pain is from the fallen arch—the fallen tarsal joint.

If there is a symptom, there must be a cause. Yet, most attention goes to the symptoms. In order to fix the symptoms properly, the cause must be located and eliminated first. Furthermore, wouldn't it be dangerous to treat the symptoms without eliminating the cause?

People hear about the heart failure, kidney failure, liver failure, and so on and know the consequences of those failures; so they do the regular checkups. But no one heard of the tarsal joint failure or the consequence of it, though we all suffer from it.

Born without the Arch?

We can see the arches in the newborn babies' feet, even though their foot bones are mostly cartilages. But, about a year later, when they start venturing out to stand and walk, their tarsal joint with super-flexible ligaments utterly flattened to the flat floor and becoming a flat foot. What can be worse than that...? So, they start their life with a body without the alignment.

However, since they cannot verbally express the falling of their tarsal joints, they instinctively compensate with the toe grabbing, tiptoeing, or pigeon toeing while learning to stand in a zigzag manner after falling several times.

This means that we, human beings, are growing, living, and dying without the alignment—unconsciously compensating all the time.

To prevent this from the start, all we need is to support the toddlers' arches with little cookie-shape orthotics. These little orthotics keep the tarsals joint from falling, so kids can stand and walk with alignment and grow with alignment. (When the toddlers use the correct little orthotics, we can see them instantly walking steadier.)

The baby's foot bones seem to grow into their own particular shapes by the age of 8 completing the tarsal joint and keep growing to reach their full size at around the age of 16 (so the size of orthotics has to be changed as the feet grow until the age of 16. After the age of 16, the size of the orthotics would not change). Some people think their feet keep growing even after the age of 16, because their shoe size gets bigger and bigger. This is one of the signs of the ever-falling tarsal joint, making the foot longer, wider, and flatter—demanding the bigger size shoes.

Growing Pain

The fallen tarsal joint can cause pain even in children's major joints, which most parents think as the "growing pains." (There was an article, "Orthotics can help Kids' Growing Pains," by the Pedorthic Association of Canada [www.pedorthic.ca] in February 2012.) Also, these days, it is common for many teenagers and young adults in their 20s or 30s experience major joint and muscle pains, even though it is too early of an age to have such problems. We now know those problems are most likely from their body moving without the alignment due to the "fallen tarsal joint."

Chapter 6

What is Walking

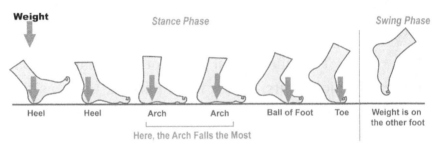

"How would you describe walking?" Most people are dumbfounded in answering this question. Some would even scoff the question saying, "What kind of question is that?" or "What do you mean? Walking is just, walking!" While there were a few philosophical answers such as, "Are you asking me . . . what is walking? That's like asking me . . . what is life." And one of my clients who was seriously limping said, "You know, life is all about walking!! I could not even approach to a girl because the way I walk . . ."

Walking is a very basic skill for our life. But no one seems to know how to describe it, more importantly, how to walk correctly. We just walk the way we have learned since we were toddlers—constantly compensating on those ever-falling, unstable tarsal joint. (It's amazing to see kids learning to stand and walk on the tilted anklebones, while simultaneously learning to compensate from that early age. Yes, babies start dealing with the harsh reality; those flat floors that do not conform to the arches of their feet.)

The mechanics of the walking cycle looks quite complicated with each foot going up and down constantly. It involves the foot, weight, and transfer. So, we can describe the walking as "the foot transferring our body weight from one place to another." And don't miss this; our body weight has to transfer through the tarsal joint to make a step.

In the walking cycle, moving a foot through the air (swing phase) is not hard at all, because the foot in the air does not carry any weight. Actually, in this swing phase, the foot gets relief momentarily from carrying the entire body weight. But the one stays on the ground (stance phase) is under the hard labor with the entire body weight (usually, more than a 100 pounds). So pressed down and relief, pressed down and relief . . . happens with each step (Yes, the relief part keeps us going).

When we think about the size of the bottom of our foot, even a humongous foot, it is a very small area to carry the entire body weight in the first place. But without the correct orthotics, we only use the heel and the ball of the foot areas (about 25% of the sole altogether) to carry our entire body weight, not utilizing the arch area (about 75% of the sole). This can flatten or dislocate the fatty tissues under the heel and the ball of the foot areas while the tarsal joint falling. So, not using the correct orthotics is abusing the foot all day by knocking down the tarsal joint against the flat surface with our entire body weight.

Usually, both tarsal joints fall with different angles and degrees. This makes one leg shorter than the other, which guarantees limping. So, most people are walking in this condition . . . limping; but people do not take this matter—our body moving without the alignment—as seriously as we should. The limping is like driving an automobile without the alignment.

How to Stand Correctly

In order to walk correctly, our body has to stand correctly first. To stand correctly, both anklebones have to be aligned first at the same height with the correct orthotics.

However, even with correct orthotics, we still can stand incorrectly. Then how to stand correctly with the correct orthotics?

With the correct orthotics, we need to stand with the body weight straight down on the anklebone, a part of the medial arch, which is designed to handle tremendous weight all day long without any issue. Easy way to achieve this is to stand with both feet at least the shoulder width apart. Then the body weight falls on the medial arch. When we stand with both feet together bring both knees together to put the body weight onto the medial arch. If the knees move even slightly to the outside, the body weight moves to the lateral arch. The lateral arch is not engineered to handle our body all day. Standing with feet apart gives out body more stability than standing with both feet together. More space between the feet, more body weight falls to the medial side.

Another thing is, however we stand, if the hips move even slightly to the backward, the body weigh goes to the heel area, which, also, is not designed to handle the entire body weight all day.

Of course, even though with the correct orthotics, our body sometimes need to stand on the lateral arch, the heel, or on the toes. But whenever possible, stand correctly with the body weight on the medial arch. If we keep standing on the lateral arch, heel or on the toes most of time, our body will give out signals with discomfort or pain in the foot or in the major joints—reminding us to stand correctly on the medial arch.

So, in order to stand correctly, two parts of our body have to work together: the tarsal joint at the bottom and the brain at the top. The tarsal joints need the correct orthotics that aligning both anklebones at the same height and the brain needs to command us to stand on the medial arch. So, even with the correct orthotics, if the brain let the body weight stand on the lateral arch, our body is not standing correctly. Without the correct orthotics, however we stand, our body cannot stand correctly.

How to Walk Correctly

With the correct orthotics, we can finally walk correctly. However, even with the correct orthotics, we still can walk incorrectly.

In order to walk correctly with the correct orthotics, the body weight should pass through the centerline of the foot that stays on the ground (stance phase).

The centerline of the foot is the highest part of the foot and the highest part of the medial arch, and it lines up from the center of the ankle to the second toe. So, when walking, bend the knee toward the second toe. This transfers the body weight through the centerline of the foot. And it's better for the body weight pass through between the first and second toe than the second and the third toe, which is close to the lateral arch.

It's good to develop a sense at the bottom of the foot as to where the weight goes. In order to feel how the body weight transfers over the foot, try the following instruction:

Stand with one foot forward as if you are about to walk; then bend the knee in front of you toward the second toe and feel how the weight transfers at the bottom of the foot. Next, bend the knee toward the big toe or the pinky toe, and feel how the weight transfers at the bottom of the foot. Is the weight transferring through the centerline of the foot, or is it off-centered? You should be able to tell if your sensory nerves are functioning properly at the bottom of the foot.

Also, walking with the feet shoulder width apart makes the body weight passes through the medial arch. This makes the catwalk incorrect walk, since the catwalk makes the body weight passes through the lateral arch.

Just remember, from the ankle toward the second toe is centerline of the foot—not toward the third toe even the third toe is in the middle.

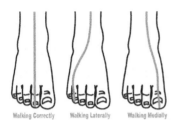

Walking Correctly   Walking Laterally   Walking Medially

Without the correct orthotics, most people have been walking with the body weight through the lateral arch unconsciously to keep the high medial arch from severe falling. These people, even with the correct orthotics, still unconsciously, walk through the lateral arch as they used to. This will eventually wear off the lateral side of the shoe bottoms and tilts the anklebones again. So, these people should train themselves to pass the body weight through the medial arch while walking. And very few people with severe knock knees who can only stand with the feet wide apart should train themselves with the knees together and bring the feet together as much possible when walking to bring the body weight between the first and second toe.

Of course, we cannot stand all the time on the medial arch or walk all the time through the medial arch. But the weight should soon come back to the medial arch before the problems develop.

If people keep standing and walking off centered, mostly on the lateral side, one side, mostly the lateral side, of the shoe bottom will wear off more than the other side and tilt the anklebone again. But good thing is, when using the correct orthotics, most likely, our body will send out signals with discomfort or pain in the foot or in the major joints as mentioned earlier. Then we can level the tilted shoe bottoms by adding the correct thickness of strips to the lower side of the shoes. Or stepping hard on the medial arch can level the shoe bottoms if the shoe bottom material is soft enough to knock it down by the by the body weight. Once the shoe bottoms are leveled, the signals—the pain or discomfort in the foot or the other joints—instantly go off.

If we walk correctly with the correct orthotics, many problems that are caused by the fallen tarsal joint can be prevented and improved.

A Walking Tip

When you walk on a rocky trail or rocky ground, look for your-arch-size rocks, and step on them right under the arch (if not using orthotics you need to look for well-rounded rocks for your feet); your feet will love those rocks pushing up against the arch where the thick muscles are. And, if you see a shallow river or stream with many smooth rocks at the bottom, take the shoes and socks off, and walk into the water stepping on those rocks under the arch as long as you can (just be careful of slippery mosses on the rocks). Afterwards, dry your feet and put the socks and shoes back on; you will have wings on your feet for a while .. !

(The word "tarsal" implies the meaning of "winged." The joint in the foot named as such implies that we fly with our feet, not with arms ... how appropriate .. !!)

Chapter 7

Orthotics, Shoes, & Socks

The orthotics, shoes, and socks all should work together for the anklebone alignment. Though, to do that, we need get the correct orthotics first.

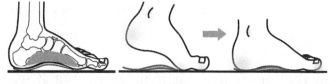 Even though the orthotics are meant to support the arch area only, most orthotics are made to go under the heel area but should not go under the ball of the foot area. So, the length of orthotics should be from right behind the ball of the foot (metatarsal heads) to the back of the heel.

The concept of orthotics, shoes, and socks for the anklebone alignment can be compared to the eyeglasses for a good vision, which is familiar to all of us. We can compare a pair of orthotics to the lenses of the eyeglasses, a pair of shoes to an eyeglass frame, and the socks or cushions that go over the orthotics to coatings on the lenses.

If the lenses are not correct, the vision cannot be clear. Similarly, if the orthotics are not correct, the anklebones cannot be aligned. As the lenses should be precisely fabricated, the orthotics should be also—even less than a half millimeter affects the alignment of the anklebones— thus, affects the even weight distribution at the bottom of the foot, just like an invisible thin dent on the eyeglass' lens affects the vision. (This means that the Creator engineered our human-machine very precisely—much more than any man-made machine.)

Even with the correct lenses, if the eyeglass frame is tilted or twisted, the vision will be impaired again. So, the frame needs be leveled. Likewise, even with the correct orthotics, if the shoe bottom is tilted or twisted, the anklebones will be misaligned again.

The coatings on the lenses are not mandatory, but if we want them, they should be the even thickness over the entire surface of the lens. If not, the vision will be affected. Likewise, socks and cushions are not mandatory for the anklebone alignment, but if we want to use them, the sock's bottom should be the same thickness throughout, and the cushion thickness should be even and cover the entire orthotics.

When our foot hurts, we try to find shoes, socks, and some nice cushions to make our foot comfortable without the correct orthotics. This is like try to get a good vision with eyeglass frames with some kind of film in them without the correct lenses. Actually, the orthotics should have been developed before the shoes, or at least alongside the shoes at the same time, just like the eyeglass frames were developed to accommodate the lenses.

To spread the words out, we need to talk about the tarsal joint and its falling, the correct orthotics and the Anklebone Alignment Test, whenever possible. Also, the orthotics with eye-catching designs surely help to draw more attention from people and they may hear this gospel for our overall body health sooner than later; and there is a saying, "faith comes from hearing . . ."

Traditional Orthotics

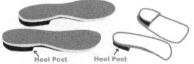

Most traditional orthotics are not attractive at all in their appearances. Usually, they are made to be thick, some even with the heel post, or the heel lift (of course some cases the heel posts are necessary), which are intimidating to look at and make them impossible to use in dress shoes or sandals. Though the heel post definitely keeps the body weight on the arch area where the weight should fall, that can be resolved by wearing the shoes with the heel higher than the front—instead of adding the heel post on the orthotics.

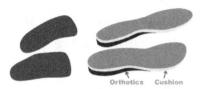

Orthotics   Cushion

There are 3/4-length and full-length orthotics. Actually, the 3/4-length orthotics are the ones enough to support the arch area. The full-length orthotics are made with cushions glued on the top of the 3/4-length orthotics. So, the front parts of the full-length orthotics are just cushions. The full-length orthotics are difficult to fit into different types of shoes. Therefore, it would be more functional to separate the orthotics and cushions; in this way we can just use the orthotics only in tight dress shoes and put the cushions over the orthotics in shoes with enough space to accommodate both.

Modern Orthotics

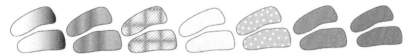

The orthotics can be made with different materials, thicknesses, shapes, and colors. In this way, they could become not only functional but also sought-after fashionable items like the shoes and the eyeglasses.

The orthotics width can be as wide as the foot or a little narrower than the foot, wide orthotics for work and sports shoes, and narrow ones for the dress shoes and high heels. Also, orthotics height can be slightly different since the tarsal joint has a slight up and down range of motion; so different orthotics support the tarsal joint at different heights within its range of motion; just make sure if the orthotics are aligning the anklebones with the Anklebone Alignment Test.

Almost every item is produced with different functions. For example, if they were shoes, there are work shoes, dress shoes, working shoes, running shoes, etc. If they were socks, thick socks, thin socks, stockings, etc. For clothes: business suits, exercise clothes, pajamas, etc. And eyeglasses, golf clubs, hats, gloves . . . you name it. Likewise, the orthotics should have developed in that manner. But they haven't. That is why those few who own orthotics most likely have only one pair (most likely got them without the Anklebone Alignment test) switching them around different shoes. It will be more functional and convenient to use different orthotics for different activities as long as they align the anklebones at the same height. Also, wearing the orthotics while taking a shower on those flat tiles would help with the fatty tissues from flattening and blood circulation at the bottom of the foot.

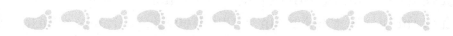

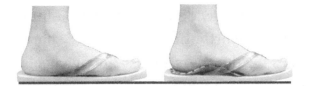 Observe the two
photos here. The foot with orthotics on the right has more
rounded shape of the heel, ball of the foot, and big toe at the
bottom, and the top of the arch is higher than the foot
without the orthotics on the left. The orthotics restore the
foot shapes by bringing the fallen tarsal joint back to where
they should be. Of course, the orthotics cannot be judged by
just looking at them—so always make sure with the
Anklebone Alignment Test.

Also, Velcro at the heel area can keep the orthotics in place
even in sandals or flip flops. They are like the nose pads of
eyeglasses. And shoe manufacturers should incorporate a
piece of the soft side of Velcro on the heel area inside the
shoes. This also can help spreading the use of the orthotics
as people may ask, "What are these Velcros for?" And
getting answers like, "Didn't you know they are for the
orthotics to align your anklebones ..?"

Observe the Shoe Bottoms

Using the correct orthotics in the tilted-bottomed shoes tilts
the anklebones again. When this happens, most likely, our
body will signal with discomfort or pain in the foot or other
major joints telling us to level the shoe bottoms. But most
people (with no idea of the importance of the shoe bottom
leveling) think that the orthotics are not working. This is
like the correct lenses in a tilted eyeglass frame, which

distort the vision. Then the frame should be adjusted—not the lenses. Just like the case with the tilted-bottomed shoes.

☆ Think about This

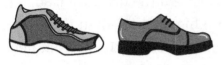 Look at the bottom of the shoes and inside of the shoes; most shoe bottoms that will step on the flat ground have arch shapes in the middle, and the inside of the shoes where our arched foot will step on is flat. Shouldn't it be the opposite? Or arch shapes inside also? Not at the outside bottom only!

Some might ask why shoe manufacturers do not make the shoes with orthotics integrated in them. It is because the orthotics cannot be generalized, since people's arch sizes are not relevant to the shoe sizes. As mentioned earlier in chapter 5, two people with the same size foot most likely have different arch sizes in length and height; so, each individual should have his/her own orthotics.

Level-Bottomed Shoes

Leveling the shoe bottom is as important as having the correct orthotics for the anklebone alignment. (The things beneath affect the alignment of the things above.)

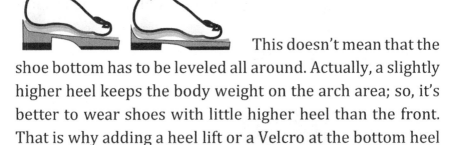 This doesn't mean that the shoe bottom has to be leveled all around. Actually, a slightly higher heel keeps the body weight on the arch area; so, it's better to wear shoes with little higher heel than the front. That is why adding a heel lift or a Velcro at the bottom heel of the orthotics would not affect the anklebone alignment.

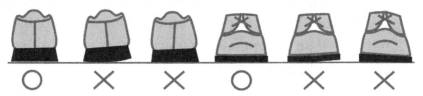

However, the shoe bottoms have to be leveled in sideways for the anklebone alignment. As mentioned earlier, even less than half millimeter thickness, which cannot be detected by the naked eyes, affect the anklebone alignment. This imperfection can be detected by the Anklebone Alignment Test. After finding the correct orthotics, put them into the shoes and do the Anklebone Alignment Test again. If the shoes bottoms are leveled, we will pass the test, if not, fail the test. Then the shoe bottoms need to be leveled by adding the correct thickness to the lower side of the inside of the shoes.

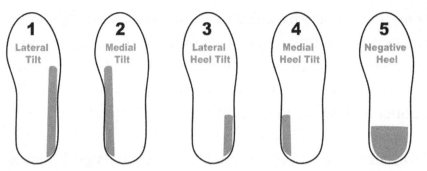

In order to level the shoes, add the correct thickness of ½"
to ¾" wide strips to the lower side of inside the shoes.

As mentioned above, shoe bottoms go off from 1 business
card thickness (which is 0.345 mm thickness) to 3 business
cards thickness—That is it. Not more than 3 business cards
thickness. So, if the shoes made us fail the Anklebone
Alignment Test, add 1 business card thickness strip and do
the test again. If fail the test again, add another strip and do
the test again. Still fail the test? Then add another one.
That's it. If the thickness is correct, we will pass the test. So,
it won't take long to find the correct thickness.

If the shoes are tilted laterally or medially (1 and 2), the
strips should be long enough for the orthotics to sit on.

Some shoes have the tilted heel (3 and 4), then add 2" long
strip to the lower side of the heel area.

For the negative heel shoes (5), add any thickness the shoes
can accommodate (usually 1/8" to 1/4" would work for
most of shoes).

Some shoe bottoms need to be leveled in two different places: the combination of 1 and 4, or 2 and 3 in the above illustration. Usually, both right and left shoes require the same levelling method. (The above illustration is for the right-side shoe, so do the same to the left shoe.)

Also, there are some shoes with slightly twisted bottoms. Surprisingly, these shoes will fail the Anklebone Alignment Test. However, those shoes can be simply fixed by twisting the shoe bottoms in the opposite direction. Then you'll be surprised by how this simple twisting makes you instantly pass the Anklebone Alignment test.

Another way to level the shoe bottoms is to use our own body weight. This method only works with the shoe bottoms made with soft material. So, if the outside (lateral side) of the shoe bottom is lower, make steps with the entire body weight on the medial side of the shoes on the hard surfaces like concrete (making steps with both feet wide apart and bring the knees together will put the body weight on the medial side of the shoes). After about 100 steps, do the Anklebone Alignment Test. if failed the test, make another 100 steps, and so on. we will pass the test if the shoe bottoms are leveled correctly. And keep trying to walk correctly through the medial arch as explained in chapter 6 to keep the shoe bottoms always leveled.

Unfortunately, about 70% of the shoes (even the brand name shoes) are produced with slightly tilted bottoms (usually laterally). So, until the shoe companies start manufacturing all the shoes with leveled bottoms, we need to level them by ourselves.

Worn-Out Shoe Bottoms

As we walk, the shoe bottoms will wear out. If we walk correctly, the shoe bottom will wear out evenly and not affect the alignment of the anklebones. But, if we do not walk correctly, usually, by standing or walking on the lateral arch, the lateral side of the shoe bottoms will wear out and misalign the anklebones again.

 Most of our shoes wear out at both lateral sides of the heel like the shoes on the left and very few at the medial side of the heel like the shoes on the right. Some people ask if these heels can tilt the anklebones. The answer is "No." This happens if we hit the ground with the lateral side of the heel right before putting the entire shoe bottom on the ground to make a step.

When the entire shoe bottom touches the ground (the stance phase in the walking cycle), the body weight doesn't go that far back of the heel. So, it doesn't affect the anklebone alignment.

Now, let's talk about some shoes that are thought to benefit our feet—but have some issues.

Double Rocker Shoes

Double rocker (bottom) shoes rock back and forth. Some materials are cut out at the bottom of the heel and the ball of the foot areas to eliminate the ground reaction force from those areas. However, this design sandwiches the arch area between our entire body weight from above and the ground reaction force from below. So, without the correct orthotics, these shoes make the tarsal joints to fall more easily than the regular shoes.

However, with correct orthotics, these shoes can be beneficial if the heel and the ball of the foot areas have some issues.

Negative Heel Shoes

Shoes with heels and lower than the front are called negative heel shoes. These negative heel shoes claim to make our body stand straighter. But what they do is tilting the body backward without aligning the anklebones. This makes the heel to carry most of the body weight all the time and hinders the circulation at the heel area—even with correct orthotics. So, these shoes make us fail the Anklebone Alignment Test. Thus, may worsen the foot condition. Hence, the negative heel shoes make no sense at all for our overall body health.

High Heels

High heel shoes definitely bring the body weight to the arch area. So, with the correct orthotics, we can wear high heels comfortably. However, if the heels are too high, the body weight will pass the arch area and all end up at the ball of the foot area, which is not desirable at all. As mentioned earlier, the body weight should be spread evenly at the bottom of the foot—including the arch area.

As we can see here, as the heel becomes higher, the arch area (the gray section where the body weight falls) becomes narrower, which is not desirable. The wider the surface, the foot can carry body weight more comfortably.

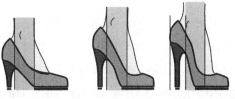

This similar illustration shows a foot in a high heel shoe. Here, we can see more clearly how the heel height affects the length of the arch area. The lower the heel, the wider the arch area. As the heel gets higher, the leg moves more forward, so the body weight falls more at the ball of the foot area, which is not desirable. So, when getting high heel shoes, make sure the heels are low enough (ideally 2 to 3 inches high) and make us pass the Anklebone Alignment Test.

Socks & Cushions

As mentioned earlier, the thickness of the bottom of socks and the cushion thickness should be the same. The socks with thick paddings on the heel and the ball of the foot areas or different knitting patterns in the middle of the arch should be avoided. Because this slight uneven thickness affects the even weight distribution at the bottom of the foot. So, to our surprise, with these socks, we will fail the Anklebone Alignment Test.

Also, the cushions need to be wide enough to cover the entire orthotics but not too wide to cause to cram up inside the shoes. This can tilt the foot and affect the anklebone alignment, and make us fail the Anklebone Alignment Test.

It's important to understand that the orthotics, shoes, socks, and cushions all work together for aligning both anklebones at the same height. Not taking all these things into consideration can negatively affect the benefit of the correct orthotics. Again, if you are not sure, always make sure with the Anklebone Alignment Test.

Chapter 8

Compensating Behaviors

Before we go any further into the Anklebone Alignment Test, we need to understand in more detail about the compensating behaviors that operate unconsciously, or rather deceivingly, in our body in an attempt to keep our body from falling due to the fallen tarsal joints. As mentioned earlier, these compensating behaviors have been programmed deeply in our body since we were toddlers. That is why many people think our body compensating is as normal. But it's not. It is from the fallen tarsal joint. These compensating behaviors keep us from testing the true physical balance of our body.

I remember asking the following questions to one of the instructors while learning how to fabricate orthotics.

I asked, "These orthotics should provide balance for our feet, right ?"
He said, "Yes."

I asked again, "Then how do we test the balance for our feet?"
He said, "Oh, we cannot do the balance test exactly on human body."

I asked again, "Why?"
He answered, "Because we are constantly moving."

I knew that "constantly moving" is the sign of our body constantly compensating—unconsciously. So, I started to observe and analyze how our body compensates on the tilted anklebones, and how it affects when testing the alignment of the anklebones.

The compensating behaviors are the defensive mechanism to counterbalance our body when there is a danger of falling. These behaviors stress the brain, use the energy, and the compensating body parts deteriorate faster. Hence, we don't want this system to be always "On" mode. It should be kicked in only when there is a danger of falling, and when there is no danger of falling the system should be turned off. But on the tilted anklebones, danger of falling is persistent. So, this compensating system is always "On" mode.

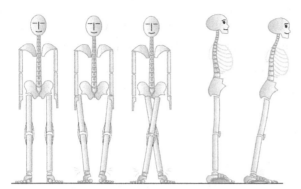

When the tarsal joint falls, it definitely falls forward and, usually, along the sideways as well. This means the tarsal joint falls in a diagonal manner. This makes the anklebone to tilt in a diagonal manner also.

Theoretically, if our body doesn't compensate on the tilted anklebones, the hip joints should fall out, or our body should fall in the direction the tarsal joint fell. However, neither the hip joints fall out, nor our body falls. Because our body compensates.

I analyzed the compensating behaviors into two categories primary and secondary compensating behaviors. Let's talk about these two.

Primary Compensating Behavior

when we are standing the tarsal joint falls by our own body weight. Then our body has to compensate to keep the body from falling. So, our body stands in a zigzag manner to keep the body from falling. I named this "Zigzag Standing" as the primary compensating behavior.

Zigzag Standing

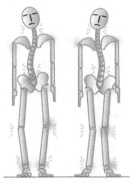

That is why we can observe this zigzag standing in most people's standing posture. This zigzag standing gets worse when we gain body weight or lift a heavy weight. Because more weight makes the tarsal joint to fall more, so tilts the anklebone more. However, we don't have control over on this zigzag standing. The only way to eliminate this zigzag standing is to align both anklebones at the same height— with the correct orthotics.

The above picture on the left depicts the tarsal joints falling laterally (supinate). This tends to tilt the anklebones laterally also. Then the legs tend to go out and compensate at the knee joints making the thighs go in to prevent the hip joint from falling out. This can develop into the bowlegs.

The picture on the right depicts when the tarsal joints falling medially (pronate). This tilts the anklebones medially also. Then the legs tend to go in and compensate at the knee joints making the thighs to go out, which can develop into the knock-knees.

If the tarsal joint falls straightforward only without tilting sideways, the legs appear to be straight, though one leg would most likely be shorter than the other, as the tarsal joint usually falls differently. Also, one thing to notice is that while the tarsal joint falls, most major joints start to go out of alignment within their normal range of motion. That is why pain doesn't start right from the beginning.

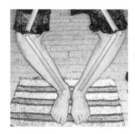 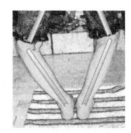 However, as time passes by, the joints could start to veer out of their normal range of motion gradually, and eventually can become like the pictures above, which causes constant pain and discomfort. This 70 years old woman's slight bowlegs became this severe after 2 years of helping her daughter's grocery store with concrete floor.

Also, when the tarsal joints fall, from the side view, the legs should lean forward, because the tarsal joint is in front of the leg bone. However, from the sideview, most young people stand with straight legs, though with one leg shorter than the other. Because they are standing on the back of the anklebone over-stretching the ligaments in front of the ankle joint.

But as the tarsal joint keeps falling, at one point, the ligaments in front of the ankle joint cannot overstretch anymore. Then the legs start to lean forward; then the thighs tilt backwards; then the hips tilt forward; then the lower back curve in (lordosis); then the upper back curves out (kyphosis); then finally, the head hangs forward.

Some cases the gravity's pull of the hanging forward head can make the entire body stoop badly. This posture waste lots of energy just to maintaining the standing posture. And may have to use a cane, the crutch, to keep the body from falling forward.

This is how the primary compensating behavior makes the body to stand in a zigzag manner—from the front view (frontal plane) and the side view (sagittal plane). These asymmetrical postures have been thought of as normal; saying, "Everybody has one leg shorter than the other," or "No one has a straight posture," or "Oh, she/he is old. So, her/his posture is like that . . ." But it is only a normal phenomenon on the tilted anklebones that is caused by the fallen tarsal joint. On the aligned anklebone, these postures most likely would not happen.

When we lift a weight with this posture, we can only lift it close to our body or has to compensate additionally.

Secondary Compensating Behaviors

A body standing with alignment from the feet up can lift a weight a little away from our body without compensating at all. But the zigzag standing body has to compensate secondarily to lift a weight a little away from our body to prevent the body from falling.

There are 3 behaviors. Let's call these behaviors as the "Secondary compensating behaviors," which operates on top of the zigzag primary compensating behavior. However, these 3 secondary compensating behaviors can be controlled by us and have to be controlled when performing the Anklebone Alignment Test for the correct result. Otherwise, we might end up with the wrong orthotics.

Those 3 secondary compensating behaviors are: the using the belly muscles, the body-tilting, and the toe-grabbing. Let's talk about these behaviors in more detail.

Using Belly Muscles

On the tilted anklebones, if we want to lift a weight a little away from our body, we cannot lift it without using our belly muscles (or core muscles). Because if we don't use the belly muscles, our body falls. A falling body cannot lift a weight.

Most people do not aware of this behavior as they are doing it unconsciously, while some people do realize using of the belly muscles but think it as normal, not knowing it is from their tilted anklebones. Either way, most people having hard time not to use the belly muscles when lifting a weight for the Anklebone Alignment Test. Also, it's hard to tell for someone who oversees the test because it's happening internally. However, we can learn to control by breathing with belly.

When we use the belly muscles, we cannot breathe with belly, so we breathe with our chest. When we are doing the Anklebone Alignment Test, we should be able to breathe with belly (the belly breathing is good fort helps the digestive system and can draw more air), and just use the arm muscles to lift the weight.

Also, if we don't use the belly muscles at all, the weight feels much lighter than lifting with the belly muscles because we don't waste the energy on the belly muscles to compensate.

Body-Tilting

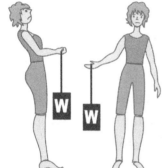

Body-tilting is another way to compensate to lift a weight a little away from our body without falling. When lifting the weight from the front, our body tilts backward and vice versa. When lifting a weight from right, our body tilt to left and vice versa. So, our body would not fall.

However, this body tilting makes our body being pulled down on both sides of the body: one side being pulled down by the actual weight and the other side by the gravity. This worsens the alignment of the body causing more damage in the joints, and the body becomes more vulnerable to injuries.

Also, Tilting the body backward puts the body weight on the heel area, and tilting the body to the right or left puts the body weight on the lateral arch. This hinders the circulation at the bottom of the foot and affects the entire body circulation since the blood vessels all connected as a whole.

Toe-grabbing

 The toe-grabbing happens when the tarsal joint falls even with just our own body weight in attempt to keep that tarsal joint from further falling. When we lift a weight, this toe-grabbing gets worse. Though, this toe-grabbing does not have much effect to keep the body from falling.

The body-tilting and the toe-grabbing behaviors are obvious and observable as they happen externally. Still, some people having a hard time controlling these compensating behaviors as these behaviors also happen unconsciously. Doing the Anklebone Alignment Test in front of a mirror can help us to see ourselves, so we can control these behaviors while looking at us in the mirror.

Two Different Standings

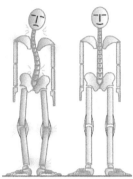

There are two different standings: standing without the alignment—false physical balance and standing with the alignment—true physical balance.

As long as we are standing, our body is balanced . . . is that right? Standing without the alignment and standing with the alignment are very different from each other. Not differentiating these two standings—or balances—could cost a fortune down the road.

Let's talk more in detail about these two different standings.

Standing without Alignment

Without the correct orthotics our body can only stand in a zigzag manner, without the alignment, from the feet up. So, this standing has the false-physical balance. This zigzag standing cannot make the centerline of the body pass through the center of the major weight-bearing joints. This means the body weight cannot be distributed evenly over the weight-bearing joints. This speeds up the joint damage.

Also, around the misaligned joint, the ligaments and muscles cannot be properly positioned, so the muscles cannot utilize their full strength. So the body becomes weak. And when this body gets jerked around in case of an accident, the body without alignment gets more damage than the body with alignment. Also, this body cannot use its full range of motion, so this body can fulfil any tasks to a certain degree only.

Standing with Alignment

With correct orthotics, our body can stand with alignment from the feet up because both anklebones are aligned at the same height nullifies the zigzag standing. So, this body has the true-physical balance. This standing makes the centerline of the body passes through the centerline of the weight-bearing joints. This can distribute the body weight evenly over the weight-bearing joints, so, minimizes the deterioration.

Also, around the aligned joints, the muscles are properly positioned. This enables the muscles to utilize their full strength and full range of motion. So becomes the body strong and makes easier for this body to fulfill any tasks to its full extend. And, when this body gets jerked around in case of an accident, the body gets less damage than the body without the alignment.

There are still so many differences in their functionalities between these two different standings: one without the correct orthotics and one with the correct orthotics. It's like analyzing the problems and benefits of an automobile running without alignment and with alignment, though the only difference is the different amount of the air in the tires.

People who practice yoga or other balance activities think they are training their body for a good balance. But, without the correct orthotics, what they are training is their brain to compensate well on the tilted anklebones. This stresses the brain and the joints not in a good way. But, with the correct orthotics, we can truly train our brain and our body muscles for the balance without compensating.

The brain is the "energy generator," and it keeps monitoring everything that is happening around us and commanding all our body activities 24/7. On the fallen tarsal joint, our entire body nerves keep sending signals to our brain to compensate constantly to keep our body from falling. This constant signaling can over-stress the brain cells and the entire nervous system. Think about the brain is doing all that work with the constant incoming signals demanding to do something to align the anklebones, which the brain cannot do by itself. This surely causes stress the brain cells and the entire nerve system. Also, this constant signaling can wear off the myelin sheath of the nerve cells. With the correct orthotics, we can free our brain from the stress that is coming from the fallen tarsal joint.

☆ Think about This

Let's say there are two simple structures with a few joints. The foundations of both structures need the proper support for its alignment. (The size of these two structures doesn't need to be the same.)

In this illustration, the structure on the left stands without the alignment due to the tilted foundation, and the structure on the right stands with alignment because the foundation is leveled with the proper support.

Now, the above two structures are wrapped with thick padding and covered with stretch fabric tubes that makes impossible to feel the joints. So, it's impossible to find out which one is which by just looking at them or touching them around. However, there is a way to find out which one is which. Can you tell . . ?

Yes, by pressing down at the top.

The one with the leveled foundation will feel solid and strong when being pressed down, while the one with the tilted foundation feels flimsy and weak. We can do the same test on human body by pressing down on someone's shoulders with both hands standing on a chair behind the person. The body stand with the correct orthotics will feel like a solid log, while the body without the correct orthotics will feel wavering and not solid. This test just gives a glimpse of the different strength between the body standing without the alignment and with alignment.

This is the basic concept of the Anklebone Alignment Test. Using the similar concept, we can do the Anklebone Alignment Test quite precisely. Let's talk about it in the next chapter.

Chapter 9

Anklebone Alignment Test

In This Chapter

Now, with the secondary compensating behaviors in mind, we can talk about the Anklebone Alignment Test (or AA test), which is the primary purpose of writing this book.

I coined the name, "Anklebone Alignment Test" for the foot balance test, thinking it would make more sense since our body stands on the anklebones, and help us to realize how critical it is to align both anklebones at the same height—for our overall body health. Also, we can clearly understand the orthotics' function should be aligning both anklebones at the same height, and there is a way to test—the "AA test." This AA test can be done one foot at a time or both feet at the same time.

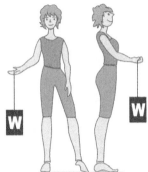

A simple way to describe the AA test is to see if the tarsal joint can handle weight without falling. In other words, to see if the anklebones are aligned or not by applying a weight on the anklebones.

A test is done by lifting a weight a little away from our body without compensating while standing on the arch. Lifting a weight little away from our body without compensating makes our body fall if the anklebones are not aligned. This fall is the indicator of the tilted anklebones.

On the aligned anklebone, the body stands with alignment from the feet up. Then the body can utilize its full strength without compensating. So, when lifting a weight for the AA test, the body with aligned anklebones can lift the weight without compensating. On the tilted anklebones, the body stands without the alignment from the feet up. Then the body cannot utilize its full strength and has to compensate all the time. So, when lifting a weight, the body will fall if not compensating. It sounds simple, but a few things should be kept in mind when doing the AA test.

1. Know how to stand on the arch, so the weight can fall on the tarsal joint.

2. Do not compensate while lifting a weight: Do not use the belly muscles, No body-tilting, No toe-grabbing. (If we know how to control these 3 secondary compensating behaviors, we can do the AA test by ourselves.)

3. The weight should be lifted at the proper distance from the body: not too close, not too far. To make the proper distance, position the elbow(s) about 3" away from the rib cage and the hand(s) about 5" below the elbow(s).

4. Lift a weight slowly. If we lift a weight quickly, most likely the compensating behaviors will kick in. Then the AA test cannot be done properly.

Standing on the Arch

Even though our body stands on the arch, most people do not know how to stand on the arch. Let's learn how to stand on the arch first.

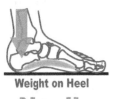
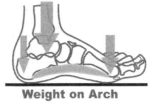
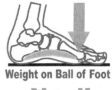

Weight on Heel	Weight on Arch	Weight on Ball of Foot
No..!!	Yes..!!!	No..!!

Anatomically, our body stands on the arch. However, mechanically, our body can stand on the heel, the ball of the foot, and, amazingly, on the toes also (these standings are like looking at the vision test chart with side eyes when doing the vision test). These areas are not engineered to carry our entire body weight for a long time. So, we don't want to stand on these areas for a long period of time—like all day.

Now, let's learn how to stand on the arch. As the hips are the center of gravity, wherever the hips go, the weight follows. Wherever the weight ends up, that is where we are standing.

So, while standing with two feet shoulder width apart, move the hips slightly back. Then the body weight goes to the heel, and we can move the ball of the foot sideways. This means we are standing on the heel—NO! the AA test CANNOT be done.

From there, slowly move the hips forward until some (not all) of the body weight hits the ball of the foot. And if we cannot move both the heel and the ball of the foot, this means we are now standing on the arch—Yes, this is the spot! The AA test CAN be done properly.

But from there, if we move the hips slightly more forward, the body weight all ends up on the ball of the foot, and we can move the heel sideways. This means we are standing on the ball of the foot—NO, the AA test CANNOT be done.

Next, let's talk about how to prevent our body from compensating behaviors.

How to Prevent Compensating Behaviors

As mentioned earlier, our body should not compensate while doing the AA test (compensating is like squinting of eyes while doing the vision test). So, we should be able to control those compensating behaviors. Though it's kind of tricky to suddenly deprogram and take control over these behaviors, since it is deeply programed in our body. But it can be done with some practice . . . or by force. Most athletes are very good at these compensating behaviors. So, pay extra attention when we do the AA test for those athletes.

First, to prevent the toe-grabbing behavior, after standing on the arch, relax the toes and lift a weight. If they keep grabbing the ground, stand with the tips of toes all lifting in the air. Do they keep insisting to grab? Then bring out about an inch high platform and stand there with the toes all hang over the front edge of it, this leaves nothing to grab onto.

Second, to prevent the body-tilting, if our body keeps tilting while lifting a weight, stand in front of a mirror and lift the weight while looking at us in the mirror. Still can't stop tilting? Then stand against a wall leaving no space between the body and the wall and lift the weight.

Third, to prevent the use of the belly muscles (the most difficult one to control), relax the belly muscles and see if we can breathe with belly. If we use the belly muscles, we cannot breathe with belly muscles. So, before lifting the weight, feel the belly area to make sure the muscles are all relaxed and can breathe with it. So, with a relaxed belly, just use the arm muscles to lift the weight while standing on the arch.

When doing the AA test, the standing body functions as a post to deliver the weight without a hindrance to the anklebones. Using the belly muscles hinders the weight from smoothly going down to the anklebone.

Remember, if we can lift a weight without the correct orthotics, we are definitely compensating.

Distance Between the Body & Weight

Also, the weight should be lifted in the proper distance. The proper distance between the body and the weight can be achieved by positioning by elbow(s) about 3" away from the rib cage and lift the hand(s) about 5" below the elbow(s) and lift the weight with that hand(s). It's like the standard distance for the vision test (6 meters or 20 feet).

Proper Distance

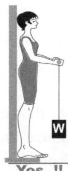

Yes..!!

To do the AA test for both feet together, position the elbows and the hands described as above and lift a weight slowly (this prevents the brain from startling and react over a fast and sudden fall of weight on the foot). While lifting, keep the hand from lifting above the elbow. Then the weight travels down to the anklebone slowly and nicely. If the hands are higher than the elbow, the weight might come too close to the body as the lifting hands pivot at the elbow toward the body.

If the orthotics are correct and align both anklebones at the same height, the body can lift the weight without compensating and be able to stay lifting the weight without falling. Without the correct orthotics, the body falls to the direction of the weight being lifted, so cannot lift the weight.

Too Close

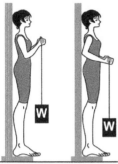

No..! No..! If the elbows stay right next to the rib cage or behind the rib cage, or the hands are above the elbows, the weight is too close to the body. Then even though the anklebones are tilted, the body won't fall. So, the AA test CANNOT be done correctly.

Too Far

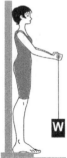

No..! If the elbows are too far from the rib cage, the weight is too far from the body. Then even with the correct orthotics, the body will fall when lifting a weight. So, the AA test CANNOT be done properly.

Once we know how to stand on the arch and the proper distance to lift a weight without compensating, the AA test can be done easily.

The amount of the weight may be determined by our muscle strength. It is recommendable to lift a weight that requires some effort to lift (about 10-15 lbs. for women, 15-20 lbs. for men). However, technically, if we don't compensate at all, especially with our belly muscles, and even if we are a very strong person, we won't be able to lift even 5 lbs. on the tilted anklebones. This means, on the tilted anklebone, in order to lift 5 lbs., we need use the belly muscles (so we cannot breathe with our belly) that is equivalent to 5 lbs.

When doing the AA test for the first time, most people compensate with the belly muscles to some degree and do not realize they are doing it so. It takes some practice not to use the belly muscles at all when lifting a weight.

Once we know how to control the compensating behaviors, especially using the belly muscles, we can do the AA test by ourselves. However, it would be good to practice with someone who knows how to do the AA test and capable of pointing out if there are compensating behaviors going on, especially with the belly muscles.

Basic Standing Test

The AA test can be done in many different postures as long as the foot touches the ground. Let's start with the "One foot at a time test." This one foot at a time AA test cannot be affected by the toe-grabbing behavior; so, we just watch 2 compensating behaviors: the body-tilting and the using the belly muscles.

One Foot at a Time Test

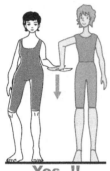

Yes..!!
After standing with both feet shoulder apart, shift the hips to the leg of the foot to be tested putting the entire body on it. The other foot should stay on the floor without carrying any weight but do not lift it from the ground. If the foot is lifted from the ground, the brain will be disturbed. Then the test cannot be done properly.

Just make sure with the other foot (without any weight) can graze over the floor. Then our body is standing on one foot.

Next, lift the hand of the foot to be tested a little lower than the elbow that is slightly away from the rib cage as described earlier. And a tester (she here) put the heel of her hand over the heel of our hand and press down slowly to the gravity direction while our hand resisting slowly up against hers. Then the weight will go down nicely to the anklebone passing through the body.

Also, she should be able to point out if we are compensating. If our body tilts to the opposite direction from her, our weight shift to the other foot. Then the test cannot be done properly. Also, remember not to use the belly muscles.

Without the correct orthotics, our body will fall without being able to resist her. With the correct orthotics, we will be able to resist with our full strength without falling or compensating.

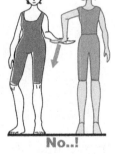

No..!   If she presses down on our hand toward our body, our body won't fall even without the correct orthotics, because the weight being applied toward our body will keep us from falling.

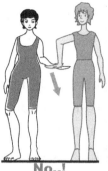

No..!   Or, if she presses down on our hand away
from our body, even with the correct orthotics, our body
will fall, because the weight being applied away from our
body will pull us and make us fall.

Both Feet Together Test

To test both feet together, we need to
stand on both feet, though make sure on the arch we are
standing (not on the heel or the ball of the foot). And
position the hands in front of us as described earlier. And
hold a shoulder length bar with both hands on each end of
it. And let her apply weight slowly on the center of the bar
straight down toward the floor as our hands resist up
against her without compensating; Don't use the belly
muscles, no body-tilting, no toe-grabbing. Without the
correct orthotics, our body will fall. With the correct

orthotics, we will be able to resist her with our full strength without falling and compensating. But be gentle not to knock her over.

Be careful to follow all the instructions. The wrong test will bring about wrong results. Then we will end up with the wrong orthotics that do not align our anklebones.

Also, we can experience the different strength. With the correct orthotics, lift a weight without using the belly muscles, and lift it using the belly muscles. The same weight feels much lighter when not using the belly muscles than using the belly muscles. Because using the belly muscles is another task and wastes the body energy.

When I do the AA test without the orthotics to anyone who looks very strong, I say to the person, "Now, this is the game of balance. I know you are much stronger than I am, but I am balanced, but you are not. So, you cannot win me . . . unless you compensate." And explain how to stand on the arch and not compensate, then, proceed with the AA test, then the person falls. And with the orthotics, I say, "Now, this is the game of strength. We both are balanced. So, I cannot win you. So~, be gentle . . ." Then the person becomes so strong and always and almost lifts me up.

Once we understand the concept of the AA test, it is rather a simple test (no involvement of chemicals or radiation), and if we know how to control the compensating behaviors, we can to the AA test by ourselves simply lifting a weight.

Do the AA Test by Ourselves

Once we can control those 3 secondary compensating behaviors at our will, we can do the AA test by ourselves. All we need is a weight to lift and follow the above instruction.

First, start with the one foot at a time AA test, and then both feet together test. With this AA test, we can find the correct orthotics, shoes, socks, cushions, or anything for our feet to make sure they are all correct for aligning our anklebones.

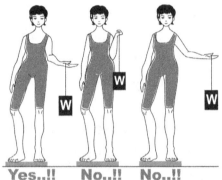

Yes..!!   No..!!   No..!!   To test one foot at a time, stand on one foot and make sure our entire body weight is on the foot to be tested and the other foot stays on the floor without any weight. And lift a weight with the proper distance with the hand as described earlier, slowly without compensating. Without the correct orthotics, our body will fall. With the correct orthotics, we will be able to lift the weight.

When lifting the weight if we tilt our body to the opposite direction, the body weight will end up on the other foot. Then the test cannot be done properly.

To test both feet together, stand on the arch, and position the hands as described earlier and lift a weight slowly with both hands without compensating, especially with the belly muscles. Without the correct orthotics, we will fall, so can't lift the weight. With the correct orthotics, we can lift the weight without compensating.

When lifting the weight, remember if our body tilts backward even slightly, the body weight will end up on the heel area. Then the test cannot be done properly.

Dynamic Posture Test

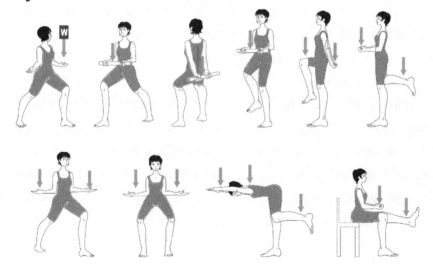

Once we mastered the basic standing AA test with total control of the compensating behaviors, we can do the AA test with all different dynamic postures: we can stand or squat down in any posture, and make sure we can maintain the posture, and simply lift a weight slowly (without compensating). With the correct orthotics, our body can utilize its full strength in any posture and can lift the weight much easier than ever, heavier weight than we used to.

Also, our body can lift weight even with a posture we never thought we can before.

Let's try this particular posture we haven't dared to lift a weight before. Because this posture involves the full faculty of the mechanical movements without sparing any movement to compensate. So, basically, with this posture, our body cannot compensate. This makes it impossible to lift weight on the tilted anklebones that requires compensation. So, our body will fall when we try to lift a weight with this posture, even though we are an expert on compensating. That is why we never thought to lift weight with this posture.

But on the aligned anklebones, our body doesn't need to compensate. So, we can lift a weight even with this posture. So, let's try . . .

First, stand with both feet **open** with a shoulder apart, and **scissor** the legs by moving on foot forward, and **bend** the knees, and **twist** the upper body over the leg in front of us. After standing still with this posture without faltering, try to lift a weight slowly, without compensating. Without the correct orthotics, our body cannot lift a weight even close our body. With the correct orthotics, we can lift a weight even a little away from our body.

And it's kind of interesting to feel that when we are about to lift a weight with this posture, our body is like thinking, "Oh, no . . . I don't think I can do this . . . with this posture . . ." but then as the strength fill the arm and the hand, we start to realize we are doing it . . !

Some emergency cases, we might have to lift a weight with this particular posture. And with the correct orthotics with the level-bottomed shoes, we can save ourselves and someone else from dangerous situations.

This means, with the correct orthotics, our wonderfully and fearfully made body machine can function fully mechanically and can do something we couldn't before.

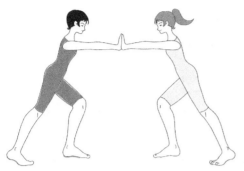

Also, experiment this push against someone's hands as illustrated here without the correct orthotics and with the correct orthotics. Pushing against someone or something with this posture puts our body weight plus the other person's or thing's pushing force right onto our tarsal joint. So. without the correct orthotics, the tarsal joint falls more misaligning our body structure worse. This makes our body to have harder time to muster up the strength. We know that the more the joints go out of alignment, the weaker the body becomes. But with the correct orthotics, the tarsal joint cannot fall. Then the body can muster up the full strength and so can push harder than ever.

Here is another posture we can try. Put one foot on a one-step stool and the other foot down on the floor with the body weight mostly on the foot on the stool. And lift a weight as the picture above. Without the correct orthotics, we won't be able to lift the weight, but with the correct orthotics, we'll be able to.

Also, when we are pressing the legs with a leg-press machine, with the correct orthotics, we can feel the knee joints moving much smoother with more strength than without the correct orthotic.

Working with many different exercise machines, we can experience the different strength of our body without and with the correct orthotics. With the correct orthotics, we can truly tell how strong our body is.

Lifting from Back Test

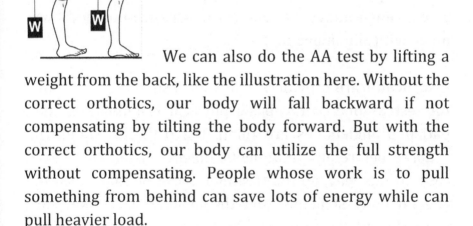

We can also do the AA test by lifting a weight from the back, like the illustration here. Without the correct orthotics, our body will fall backward if not compensating by tilting the body forward. But with the correct orthotics, our body can utilize the full strength without compensating. People whose work is to pull something from behind can save lots of energy while can pull heavier load.

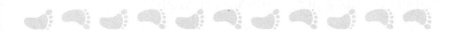

Basic Physical Test

Even though we do not have any symptoms, we do the basic health tests periodically to prevent any unpleasant surprises: a blood pressure test to prevent a heart attack, or a blood sugar level test to prevent diabetes, and, etc., etc. Likewise, the AA test should be done periodically to prevent the problems that are caused by the fallen tarsal joint.

We can do this AA test at home before heading out to school or for work to check everything we put on our feet (the orthotics, shoes, and socks) are working together for the anklebone alignment. Especially, for the shoe bottom levels. Because even with the correct orthotics, if we don't walk correctly for a while, the shoe bottoms can wear off and tilt the anklebones. Then we can level the shoe bottoms too as explained in chapter 7. All we need is a weight near the front door or apply weight on each other's hands while standing as explained above. So, we can make sure our body will move with alignment all day.

Also, healthcare providers at any level should perform this AA test as one of the basic physical examinations. If a patient's anklebones are tilted, the orthotics should be ordered before any treatments, unless it is an emergency case. In this way, all the treatments can be done with the aligned body structure and the healings can take place properly with the aligned body structure. Otherwise, all the treatments will be done without the alignment, and the healings will take place without the alignment.

I hear people say "I used to have back pain (or other areas), but it's all healed. Now my knees (or other areas) are hurting." Then I say, "Yes, your back is healed but not with alignment. This means most likely your back lost some of the range of motion. Now, your knees are compensating more than ever due to your back not being able to compensate like before, and your tarsal joints keep falling . . . until you use the correct orthotics."

This is how our posture changes, as time passes by. Look at the people with foot deformities, bowlegs (or knock knees), body lean to one side, or hunched back; it happens gradually little by little as our body alleviates the discomfort or pain and does some fixing and healing on its own without the alignment, all the while the tarsal joints keep falling.

Chapter 10

Fallen Tarsal Joint & Foot Deformities

In This Chapter
- Hammer Toes
- Mallet Toes
- Claw Toes
- Overlapping Toes
- Morton's Toe
- Pigeon Toes
- Flat Foot
- Splay Foot
- Duck Feet
- Bunion & Tailor Bunion
    - Conditional Bunion
    - Structural Bunion
- Calluses
- Pump Bump
- Protrusion of the 5th Metatarsal Root
- Floating Bones
- Coalition of the Tarsal Bone

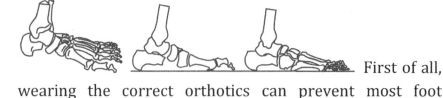 First of all, wearing the correct orthotics can prevent most foot

deformities as they are developing with each step as the tarsal joint falls with each step.

The fallen tarsal joint puts the entire foot bones out of alignment and stretches the skin of the sole. However, the foot deformities are more noticeable on the toe areas than the arch area, even though they are starting from the arch, the tarsal joint, going out of alignment. (Some put screws in the tarsal joint attempting to align the foot bones.)

Some people think they are born with foot deformities. But unless presented at birth, most foot deformities develop as the tarsal joint falls with each step. The hereditary factors are the arch height and the muscle characteristics as mentioned in chapter 4 and the shoe types we usually wear.

The first sign of the fallen tarsal joint is the tips of the toes grabbing the ground. The regular length toes usually look normal from the top of the foot with straight looking toes, but the long toes have bent joints from the top of the foot.

But from the bottom, we can see some or all the tips of the small toes are close to the ball of the foot, even the short toes. This toe grabbing gets worse as the tarsal joint falls more as time passes by. Many elderly people have the small toes all jammed up to the ball of the foot area. The foot with tight ligaments/muscles are prone to have more severe toe grabbing than the foot with the flexible ligaments/muscles. This toe grabbing shortens the toe flexor tendons that run at the bottom of the toes.

Now, let's start with hammer toes . . .

Hammer Toes

The hammer toes develop as the second joints from the tips of the toes (proximal phalangeal joints) bend to grab the ground.

(I was sure the tarsal joint was falling from ancient times, more severely after Romans paved the road with stones. So, I visited museums to see the feet from the antient paintings and sculptures. There I saw almost every bare foot or sandal clad foot has the hammer toes. And from some sculptures I could see the bottom of the foot with the small toes all close to the ball of the foot—the toe grabbing, the sign of the fallen tarsal joint.)

Mallet Toes

The mallet toes develop as the first joints from the tips of the toes (distal phalangeal joints) bend to grab the ground.

Claw-Toes

The claw-toes are advanced stage of the mallet-toes. Because as the tarsal joint keeps falling more and more with each step, the mallet-toes grab the ground more fiercely with each step and eventually can become the claw-toes. For this reason, this deformity can be seen more in older people's feet.

Treatment: The correct orthotics prevents the tarsal joint from falling and bring the fallen tarsal joint back to where it should be. Then the toes don't need to grab the ground anymore. So, the condition can get better as time passes by. Massaging the tightened toe flex tendons at the bottom of the toes (flexor digitorum tendons) can stretch and soften the tendons little by little, then the toes can become straighter little by little.

Overlapping Toe

When the tarsal joint falls, the toes tend to go up. Then they grab the ground to stabilize themselves while trying to keep the tarsal joint from further falling. When this happens inside of narrow-toe-box shoe while the toes are all cramped together, the toes can grab onto whatever is on the way. Usually, the second toe, which is probably in the most unstable condition due to falling from the highest part of the arch, tend to grab any toes next to it (usually the big toe).

Treatment: The correct orthotics relax the toes by keeping the tarsal joints from falling. Massaging between the overlapped toes and using a toe spacer between the toes can help to separate the toes.

Morton's Toe

When the tarsal joint falls through the centerline of the foot (the highest part of the arch) toward the second toe, the second toe gets pushed forward more than the other toes and can become longer than the other toes. This misaligns the head of the metatarsal bones at the ball of the foot area overstretching the ligaments and all the soft tissues. This, also, can pinch the nerves and blood vessels between the misaligned heads of the metatarsal bones. This can make the ball of the foot area very sensitive and can trigger the pain when standing and walking.

Treatment: The correct orthotics can align the foot bones, then the ligaments, nerves, and blood vessels can position themselves to the proper position without pulling and squeezing. Now, with the orthotics, the arch area can handle most of the body weight releasing the ball of the foot area from the excessive body weight. Massaging the foot gently can speed up the recovery as it further helps the blood circulation.

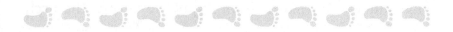

Pigeon-Toes

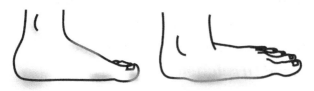

The pigeon-toes happen while attempting to prevent the high medial arch from falling. Some people, especially, kids unconsciously bring the toes medially and curl up the medial arch while standing and walking. This can eventually develop into the pigeon-toes. This also puts the body weight on the lateral arch, which is not good either.

Treatment: Use the correct orthotics and practice to walk correctly by placing the foot straight in front of the leg and transferring the body weight through the medial arch.

Flat Foot

As mentioned earlier the flat foot happens as the tarsal joint falls completely to the ground. Kids' tarsal joint with still-growing-flexible ligaments usually falls like this. But after their ligaments start to tighten up as they grow, the arch might appear a little bit, but their tarsal joints are still all out of alignment. People born with flexible ligaments are prone to have this flat foot, even though they are born with high arch. As mentioned earlier no one is ever born with flat foot unless it's a birth defect.

Treatment: The correct orthotics align the tarsal joint recovering the arch, and we can strengthen all the weakened ligaments and muscles under the arch area by exercising the toes by flexing up and down without moving the ankle joint.

Splay Foot

This splay foot can be called as a "Pancaked foot" as the entire foot spreading out as a pancake. When the tarsal joint falls freely in a wide space without the toes grabbing the ground, the metatarsal bones can really spread out leading the toes all spread out as well. People with flexible muscles who like to wear flip flops or wide toe-box shoes tend to develop this foot deformity. This splay foot usually accompanies the flat foot.

Treatment: Use the correct orthotics and bind the arch area including the ball of the foot with elastic band, such as kinetic tapes, to bring the overstretched ligaments and tendons back together. When binding the foot, remember not to block the blood circulation by binding too tight.

Duck Feet

When the tarsal joint falls medially the muscles and ligaments in the medial side of the foot can be overstretched. Then the front part of the foot tends to go outward and slowly developing into the duck feet.

Treatment: Use the correct orthotics and stand and walk correctly putting the foot straight from the ankle. And exercising the overstretched ligaments and tendons in the medial side of the foot by flexing the medial arch up toward medially may speed up the correction of this foot deformity.

Bunion & Tailor's Bunion

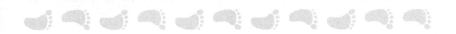

The bunion is a bump at the side of the big toe, and tailor's bunion is a bump at the side of the pinky toe. Both develop in narrow toe box shoes as both sides of the ball of the foot rubbing the shoe wall with each step as the tarsal joint falls with each step all day (about 2,500 times a day per foot if we walk about 5,000 steps a day).

As the arch at the big toe side (medial arch) is higher than the arch at the pinky toe side (lateral arch), the big toe side elongates more when the tarsal falls, so the big toe side rubs against the shoe wall more severely than the pinky toe side. Therefore, the bunion is more likely to happen than the tailor's bunion.

People with flexible muscles and high arches are prone to develop this foot deformity when they wear narrow-toe-box shoes. But even people with tight muscles can develop a bunion in their old age as their tarsal joint falls easily due to the over-stretched and weakened plantar ligaments.
There are two types of bunions: Conditional bunion and Structural bunion.

Conditional Bunion

The conditional bunion is just a bump or callous buildup at the side of the big toe while the big toe remains somewhat straight. This happens as the tarsal joint falls in not-so-narrow toe-box shoes.

Treatment: The correct orthotics realign the fallen tarsal joint and keep the joint from falling. This stops the bunion from getting worse and can start getting better. Massaging the callused area with moisturizing cream can soften the callus.

Structural Bunion

The structural bunion happens as the tarsal joint falls inside of narrow-toe-box shoes. In those shoes, the toes are all squeezed into the narrow toe box with no room in front for the elongated foot to go as the tarsal joint falls with each step. Then the joints at the side of the big toe bends out overstretching the ligaments between the

1st and 2nd metatarsal heads and forming the structural bunion.

Also, the side of the big toe rubbing against the shoe wall can hardens the skin to develop callus, or if the material of the inside shoe is like plastic material, the skin at the big toe may stick to the wall, then the skin there can become thin and rea as the head of the 1st metatarsal rubbing the inside the skin against the shoe wall. The rubbing force from the entire body weight can even stretch the shoe walls out misshaping the shoes as well.

Treatment: The correct orthotics realign the tarsal joint and keep it from falling. This instantly stops the bunion from getting worse and the condition can get better. And binding the ball of the foot area with elastic bands can bring the overstretched ligaments between the heads of the metatarsal bones back together.

Many people think the hammer toes and bunions as hereditary, but they are the consequences of the fallen total joint. So, even a bunion is removed by a surgery, it most likely comes back again as the remaining tarsal joint continues to fall with each step after the surgery. So, using the correct orthotics can prevent the bunion from happening and from recurring after the surgery.

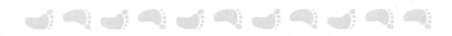

Calluses

Without the orthotics, the entire body weight only goes to the heel, ball of the foot, and toe areas. This weight hinders the circulation in these areas. In addition to that, these areas have to bear the frictions against the bottom of the shoe as the arch stretches with each step as the tarsal joint falls all day. This can cause callus (thick, harden layer of skin) build up in these areas. We can see this callus build up as one of our body's protecting systems to prevent the skin from tearing apart from constant pressure or friction.

Energetic children wearing sneakers most of time and jumping around all day can build up calluses even on the top of their foot as the fluctuating arch creates friction against the ceiling of the shoes.

Treatment: Using the correct orthotics keep the tarsal joint from falling. So, no more fluctuating at the top of the foot or friction at the bottom of the foot. And the body weight can be spread evenly throughout the bottom of the foot, including the arch area; this helps the blood circulation, so, the calluses can diminish gradually. File off the callused area and applying moisturizing cream can help.

Pump Bump

When the tarsal joint falls with each step, the back of the heel pumps up and down with each step. This action creates friction on the back of the heel against the back of the shoe (the heel counter) and eventually can cause the callous build-up there. This happens more with high arched foot with flexible muscles. (This deformity is also known as the Haglund's deformity.)

Treatment: The correct orthotics keeps the tarsal joint from falling. Then the heel cannot pump up and down, so eliminates the friction at the back of the heel. Then the condition stops getting worse and can get better little by little.

Protrusion of the 5th Metatarsal Roots

This protrusion of the root of the 5th metatarsal bone is another noticeable deformity of the arch area beside the flat foot due to the fallen tarsal joint. This little bump in the middle of the lateral arch indicates the flattening of the 5th metatarsal bone on the ground as the lateral arch falls severely. Then the wide part of the root of the 5th metatarsal bone lays flat on the ground pushing the skin out right there. This is how this protrusion happens. We can see this deformity in young kids' feet, like from 7–8 years old feet.

Treatment: As the correct orthotics bring the tarsal joint in alignment, the 5th metatarsal bones can reposition to its proper angle. Then the protrusion can be prevented and be diminished.

Floating Bones

Some foot x-ray images show some small floating bones. This could have happened as the tarsal joint severely falls when kids jumping around while the bone are still growing with lots of cartilage. Then the foot bones are knocking each other chipping off small pieces of the soft bones and they float around the joints and calcified.

Treatment: The correct orthotics keep the tarsal joint from falling, even kids jump off from the highest places. This can prevent the foot bones from knocking off each other. Theb the foot bones cannot be chipped off.

Coalition of the Tarsal Bones

The coalition of the tarsal bones is fusing of two or more of tarsal bones. This can happen when kids jump around a lot, their foot bones with lots of cartilage knocking each other severely with the force of their entire body weight. This force can fuse the soft bones together while the small tarsal bones are tightly clustered without the alignment. This fusion usually involves the anklebone, heel bone, and the navicular bone.

Treatment: Using the correct orthotics keep the tarsal joint in alignment. This prevents the foot bones from knocking each other and the foot bones can grow with alignment. So, the coalition of the tarsal bones most likely won't happen. Once the tarsal bones are fused, the orthotics would not separate them but can help eliminating the pain caused by the coalition.

Using the correct orthotics and walk correctly can prevent and improve all the above foot deformities.

Observe toddlers' feet while standing or walking; their toes are grabbing the ground with their arches flat on the floor. This means toddlers' feet are already in the process of deforming. Some smart kids may walk on their toes (toe-walking) or pigeon-toeing. And some super-smart kids already perceive what is going to happen to their tarsal joint on the flat floor, so stubbornly refuse to even stand on the flat floors. These signs are the kid's ways of expressing, "Mommy, daddy, my tarsal joint is falling. Do something, please . . ."

Even a little support can keep the kids' tarsal joint from collapsing. When we support the toddlers' arches accordingly, we can see them walking steadier instantly without staggering or falling. This also makes the kids' feet and body to grow with alignment.

Chapter 11

Fallen Tarsal Joint & Aching Foot

In This Chapter
- Plantar Fasciitis
- Heel Spur
- Metatarsalgia
- Neuroma
- Gout
- Ulcer
- Pain around the Heel
- Charcot Foot
- Sever's Disease
- Kohler's Disease
- How to Strengthen the Foot Muscles

Fallen tarsal joint disengages the entire foot bones; then all the foot ligaments, tendons, muscles, and nerves either over-stretch or get pinched by the misaligned joints. Also, without the correct orthotics, the body weight only goes to the heel, the ball of the foot, and the toes. This can cause foot pain. Wearing the correct orthotics can bring all those soft tissues to their proper position while spreading the body weight evenly at the bottom of the foot, so can prevent and improve the foot pain.

Let's start with plantar fasciitis.

Plantar Fasciitis

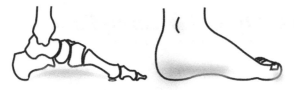

Plantar fasciitis is the inflammation of the plantar fascia ligament that runs under the tarsal joint from the front of the heel bone to the back of the metatarsal heads. When the tarsal joint falls with each step, this ligament overstretches with each step and sometimes can even tear apart causing inflammation and pain.

We all should assume that our plantar fascia ligament has some degree of inflammation. we just don't realize it until the pain certainly starts in the morning as we take the first step out of bed or stand up after sitting for a while.

There is a reason why pain starts after the foot seems to have a plenty of rest. When the foot is resting without any weight on it, the tarsal joint doesn't fall. Then the connective tissues start to heal the damaged ligament. But when we stand up again without the correct orthotics the tarsal joint falls again overstretching the ligament and tearing apart the partially healed ligament causing the "Ouch!". As we keep walking the ligament keeps overstretching with each step, then pain may subside as the tearing of the partially healed ligament is over.

However, at night when we go to bed, the healing happens again and the next morning when we make the first step out of bed, and again, the partially healed plantar fascia ligament tears apart shooting out the pain again. So, this healing and tearing cycle keeps repeating weakening the plantar fascia ligament. When the inflammation gets severe, the walking can become very difficult due to the pain. Also, this healing and tearing cycle can cause scar tissue build-ups on the ligaments that can be palpated as bumpy knots at the bottom of the arch.

Sometimes, even toddlers cry out at night holding their feet. These kids may have been born to have tight muscles. So, during the day while walking kids' tarsal joints completely fall to the ground overstretching the plantar fascia ligament and become inflamed at night causing pain.

Treatment: The correct orthotics realigns the fallen tarsal joint and keep the joint from falling. Then the proper healing of the plantar fasciitis can take place. Immersing the feet into hot and cold water alternately helps the blood circulation, which can speed up the healing. Flexing the toes up and down can strengthen the plantar fascia ligament.

(Blood is the actual healing agent delivering the oxygen and nutrients in and the waste out. So, it should be able to flow without any hinderance. Distributing the weight evenly at the weight-bearing surface, massaging, and applying hot and cold packs or immersing into hot and cold water can help the blood circulation. When applying hot and cold pack or water, wait until the part being treated all relaxed with hot pack or water and al contracted to cold pack or water for maximum pumping of the blood.)

Some people do plantar release surgery, which by cutting the part of the plantar fascia ligament to eliminate the pain from overstretching. But this makes the tarsal joint to fall more easily worsening the structural problems all over our body down the road. And the cortisone shots ruin the healing process by damaging the ligament forever.

Heel Spur

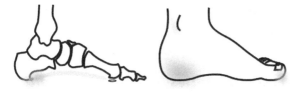

When the tarsal joint falls, the heel bone rolls backward. Then the sharp edge at the bottom front of the heel bone faces the ground. Then the ligament attached to that part pressed down by the weight while being overstretched with each step. This can eventually cause the ligament to tear apart from the heel bone. Then the uric acid lingering around that area caught into the roughly damaged surfaces of the bone and the ligament and absorbs calcium from the bone or ligament, and, as time passes by, it grows like a bone in a little thorn shape at the bottom front of the heel bone. This is the heel spur. Walking on this heel spur can be very painful. Also, we can see this heel spur as the second stage of the plantar fasciitis.

(Uric acid is the waste product of nutrients that appears as powder-like crystals in various shapes and sizes. This uric acid should be flushed out of our body through urine. However, at the bottom of the foot where usually has poor blood circulation, this uric acid can accumulate more than other parts of our body.)

Treatment: The correct orthotics bring the heel bones to the proper position by realigning the tarsal joint and spread the body weight evenly at the bottom of the foot including the arch area. This relieves the heel from too much weight bearing. Then the pain can subside and even disappear.

Metatarsalgia

Without the correct orthotics, the body weight only goes to the heel, ball of the foot and the toe area while the tarsal joint falls. Then the metatarsal heads in the ball of the foot area go out of alignment overstretching the ligaments in between them while the fatty tissues under the ball of the foot flattens out by the weight. With this condition, bearing the weight more than its portion can inflame the area and trigger the pain.

Treatment: The correct orthotics realigns the fallen tarsal joint. This realigns the metatarsal heads also. And now, with the orthotics, the arch part can carry big portion of the body weight relieving the ball of the foot area from being out of alignment and carrying too much weight. Then the pain can subside and even disappear as the metatarsalgia being healed with alignment.

Neuroma

When the tarsal joint falls, the metatarsal arch goes alignment too. Then the foot nerves between the metatarsal heads can be pinched between them, especially in tight shoes. Keep walking with this condition can damage the nerves and eventually can cause pain.

Treatment: The correct orthotics aligns the tarsal joint. This realigns the metatarsal bones as well releasing the nerves from being pinched and the proper healing can take place with alignment. Applying warm and cold packs alternately over the painful area can help the circulation and speed up the healing process.

Gout

As the tarsal joint falls with each step, the cartilages, and the ligaments at the side of the big toe where the most friction happens against the shoe wall can get damaged. Then the floating uric acid around the area can agitate the damaged cartilage and ligaments and can cause inflammation and pain.

Treatment: the correct orthotics keeps the tarsal joint from falling. This eliminates the friction from the side of the big toe, so stops the further damage in the cartilages and ligaments. Elevating the foot and gentle massage around the affected area can disperse the uric acid away from the damaged area. This can help reducing the pain while the healing takes place.

Ulcer

An ulcer is an open sore that usually develops at the ball of the foot, heel, and 5th metatarsal root areas where the weight tends to go when there is no correct orthotics. Especially, people with diabetes tend to develop these ulcers when the foot nerves malfunction and become numb. While the foot has the functional nerves, the foot tries to move around the weight from the damaged area to alleviate the weight that causing the pain. But, with the numb nerves, no pain even though the wound is severe and becomes an open sore.

Treatment: The correct orthotics distribute the body weight evenly throughout the bottom of the foot, thus, helps the blood circulation. Massaging around the ulcers and cushy cushions over the orthotics can improve circulation, so, can speed up the healing process.

Pain around the Heel

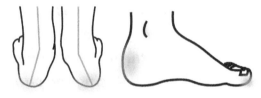

When the tarsal joint falls, the heel bone tilts pulling and stressing the ligaments and tendons around the heel bone. Then the inflammation can happen in the ligaments and tendons around the heel bone and can cause pain.

Treatment: The correct orthotics aligns the tarsal joint. This keeps the heel bone from tilting. Then the ligaments and tendons around the heel bone go back to their proper position without getting pulled. Exercise the ligaments and tendons by moving the foot around the ankle joint gently, and massaging the area helps the healing process with better blood circulation.

Charcot Foot

When the tarsal joint falls with each step, the foot nerves can be weakened by overstretching, twisting, and pinching. The weak nerves mean weak muscles, as the nerves deliver the strength to the muscles. This causes the tarsal joint to fall more easily. Then the nerves become weaker; then the tarsal joint falls even more weakening the foot muscles worse.

This cycle of damaging the foot nerves and muscles continues until the tarsal joint's complete collapse putting all the foot bones totally out of alignment. This damages the foot nerves severely causing many complicated problems. This is the condition of the Charcot foot. People with this condition have very poor balance. So, they can fall easily and get hurt. People with flexible ligaments tend to have this problem.

Treatment: Using the correct orthotics is critical to prevent and improve this dire foot problem. Massaging the foot gently and using cushions over the orthotics can better the blood circulation and exercise the muscles by flexing the toes up and down and moving the foot around the ankle joint can help further circulation, then the condition can be improved.

Sever's Disease

This is the Inflammation of the growth plate (soft sponge-like part of the bone) of the heel bone.

It usually happens to relatively active children from age 9 to 14 while their bones are still growing. When the tarsal joint falls, the heel bone tilts. This pulls the Achilles tendon that is embedded to the back of the heel bone. In some cases when the tarsal joint falls severely, instead of the tendon being tearing apart from the bone, the growth plate pulls apart causing inflammation and pain on the growth plate.

Treatment: The correct orthotics align the tarsal joint and keep the heel bones from tilting. Then the healing takes place. Binding the back of the heel bone to the front of the ankle area with flexible tape (like kinesiology tape) can tighten the growth plate in place for proper and faster healing.

Kohler's Disease

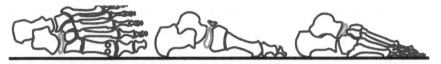

The Kohler's disease is the navicular bone not growing into its normal shape and size.

The navicular is the last foot bone to be calcified. It is located between the anklebone and the 3 cuneiforms. When the tarsal joint falls, the space for this still-growing navicular gets jammed between the already calcified anklebone and the 3 cuneiforms. This tight space and poor blood circulation hinders the navicular's normal growth leaving the navicular bone much thinner and weaker. When the tarsal joint falls severely as kids jump down from high place, the impact can even break this poor navicular bone.

Treatment: The correct orthotics keeps the tarsal joint from falling. So, all the foot bones, including the slow-growing navicular bone, can grow into their particular shapes with alignment and good circulation.

The correct orthotics can prevent all the above problems, and the existing problems can start to improve and heal properly with the alignment.

Though, some people think the orthotics as crutches. No, they are NOT. . !! They are the essential device for the alignment of our body from the feet up. As mentioned earlier, the support was there, the soft soil, when we were walking with barefoot on the soft soil. But now, on the flat floors, we need man-made supports, the orthotics. Then our body can move with alignment from the feet up as long as we live.

How to Strengthen the Foot Muscles

There are many different machines to exercise different parts of our body. But there is no machine to exercise the foot. Shouldn't the foot be healthy and strong first to hold up the rest of the body properly for exercise .. ?

We can keep our foot healthy by just walking correctly with the correct orthotics with level bottomed shoes just like we can keep our body healthy just by walking. However, if we like to strengthen the foot by exercising, we can do so while sitting or lying down on our bed. To exercise the foot, the foot should not be at work, which means the foot should not carry our body weight.

So, while sitting or lying down, lift the foot (or feet) in the air in a straight position from the leg, and flex the toes up and down without moving the ankle joint. This can strengthen all the foot ligaments, tendons, and muscles in the correct manner. Start with slow and gentle flex, and as the foot becomes stronger, the toes can be flexed with more force and as forceful as we can. If there is accumulated waste at the arch area due to the poor circulation, cramps might happen at the arch area while flexing the toes. Then lift the feet high up and massage the arch area to help the circulation going. And resume flexing the toes gently again.

Always use the orthotics when standing and walking. We should consider the orthotics as an organ. Its function? Aligning both anklebones at the same height, which can spread the weight throughout the bottom of the foot.

Remember, if we don't use orthotics, our foot starts to become weak; by hindering the blood circulation at the bottom of the foot and forcing the foot into work with all the foot joints out of alignment.

Chapter 12

Problems Above the Foot

The fallen tarsal Joint causes problems above the foot, as the fallen tarsal joint puts the entire body structure out of alignment. Let's start with the Achilles tendonitis.

Achilles Tendonitis

As the tarsal joint keeps falling with each step all day, the heel bone keeps tilting and twisting with every step torquing the Achilles tendon. This can eventually overstretch the tendon and cause inflammation and pain.

Treatment: The correct orthotics keeps the tarsal joint in alignment. Then the heel bone is not going to twist. This instantly keeps the Achilles tendon from twisting and torquing and relieving the pain.

Shin Splint

The shin muscle (tibialis anterior) is imbedded to the front of the shin bone (or leg bone). This muscle becomes a tendon as it goes down and passes the ankle joint and the tarsal joint and attached to the root of the first metatarsal bone. So, when the tarsal joint falls, this tendon is pulled down pulling the entire shin muscles. When running, the pulling gets worse as tarsal joint falls more than while walking; then this shin muscle can be pulled off from the shin bone and cause pain in front of the leg bone.

Treatment: The correct orthotics keeps the tarsal joint from falling; thus, the shin muscle would not be pulled down. So, just wearing the correct orthotics can eliminate the pain relatively quick.

Usually, the pain from Achilles tendonitis and shin splint disappears instantly by using the correct orthotics. Also, once we train ourselves to walk correctly through the centerline of our foot, our body can run faster than before without damaging the tarsal joint.

Knee Problems

When the tarsal joint falls, the knee joint goes out of alignment. Then all the ligaments and tendons around the knee joints are pulled and twisted in an incorrect manner, and the cartilages and menisci between the knee joint get stressed out by uneven weight distribution. This eventually damages the knee joint in and around with inflammation and become arthritic down the road. Also, the kneecaps can be pulled and dislocated.

Treatment: The correct orthotics can align the knee joint, then all the ligaments and tendons around the knee joint can work with alignment, and the even weight distribution between the joint can help the cartilages and menisci to heal properly with alignment. Also, massaging around the knee joint can speed up the healing.

There are quite a few ligaments and tendons around the knee joints that would be affected negatively by the fallen tarsal joint: the anterior/posterior cruciate ligaments, medial/lateral collateral ligaments, medial/lateral meniscus, patella ligaments, quadriceps tendon, hamstring tendon, and iliotibial band.

Many people are suffering from the knee joint problems not knowing both anklebones should be aligned first with correct orthotics to stop further damage, and then the proper healing can take place with alignment.

Leg Length Discrepancy

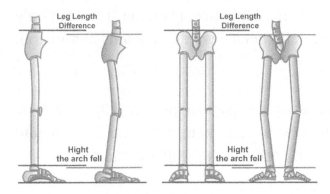

The diagram here shows how the fallen tarsal joint affects the leg length as both tarsal joints fall in different degrees and angles. We measure the leg length from the floor to the top of the hip bone, the iliac crest. Therefore . . .

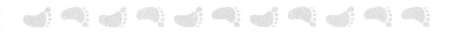

The leg length = the foot height (= the anklebone height from the floor) + leg height + the thigh height + the hip height.

The fallen tarsal joint tilts the anklebone making the leg, thigh, hip bones all stand without the alignment in a zigzag manner. We know anything that stands without the alignment stands shorter than when it stands with alignment. So, all these bones standing without the alignment shortens the overall leg length much shorter than the height of the tarsal joint fell. And as both tarsal joints falling differently makes one leg shorter than the other. The leg standing on the more-fallen tarsal joint stands shorter than the leg standing on the less-fallen tarsal joint. This, unquestionably, tilts the hipbones. Then the spine can only stand without the alignment, which shortens the overall body height.

With the correct orthotics, we can get our height back by standing straighter with alignment from the feet up, and some people feel they are standing taller instantly.

Very few people are actually born with or have one leg shorter than the other for some reason. In that case, after aligning the anklebones at the same height, add a heel lift under the orthotics or the whole foot lift of the shorter leg to make both leg length the same. Then the spine can stand with alignment.

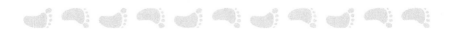

The height of the heel lift or the whole foot lift can be precisely measured by the two feet together AA test.

Some people put a heel lift under the heel of the shorter leg without the correct orthotics in attempt to make both leg length the same to relieve the back pain, or a cushion under the painful heel. But, this might relieve the back pain momentarily, but without the correct orthotics, this gives the tarsal joint more room to fall . . !! So, eventually, the body will have more problems down the road as the tarsal joint can fall more severely.

Another way some people attempt to make different leg length the same is adding thickness at the whole shoe bottom of the shorter leg. This can level the hip bones sideways, but they are still in a tilted forward position. Also, this puts the entire leg into shorter space. This stresses the joints in between and makes the tarsal joint to fall more easily, thus, invites more problems down the road.

Treatment: Simply aligning both anklebones at the same height with the correct orthotics can make the leg length the same instantly. Then the hip bones can sit with alignment.

Herniated Disc

The herniated disc is another simple alignment problem. The fallen tarsal joint definitely tilts the hip bones forward and along the sideways. This tilts the Lumbar 5 (L5) forward making the lower back to curve in (lordosis). Then the back of all the lumbar vertebrae squeezes the back part of every disc, and the front spaces of the vertebrae open up. This can cause the discs squeeze out from the back of the spine or slide down from the front of the spine and become herniated discs.

Treatment: As the correct orthotics realign the hip bones. Then the spine can stand with alignment. This can free the discs from being squeezed and sliding out, so prevents the herniated discs. Even after the surgery, with the correct orthotics, the proper healing can take place with alignment.

Scoliosis

Most people, even kids, have some degree of scoliosis as most people have the fallen tarsal joint, both differently. So the hip bones all tilted diagonally. The spine standing on the diagonally tilted hips can only stand with some curvature and twist and causes one shoulder blade (scapula) higher than the other side.

If the tarsal joint falls forward only (though this rarely happens), the hip bones only tilt forward. This makes the spine look straight from the front view, but from the side view, the lower back caves in (lordosis) and the upper back bulges out (kyphosis). When this gets severe, the hunchback happens.

Treatment: the correct orthotics systematically align the hip bones. Then the spine can gradually straighten up by itself. If it's severe, wearing a spine brace can speed up the correction.

As mentioned earlier, the alignment must be checked in a standing posture from the feet up, just like the alignment of every standing structure starts at the bottom. So, the number of the vertebrae should start from the bottom, not from the top to bottom. So, the Lumbar 5 becomes the Lumbar 1, Lumbar 4 becomes Lumbar 2, and the number gets bigger as it goes up. This might help people to see the alignment starts at the bottom, from number 1, like the other structures—not from the top.

Then people would not attempt to align our body structure in a lying down position, which goes out of alignment right after we stand up and walk few steps without the correct orthotics.

Scoliosis is one of the symptoms of the fallen tarsal joint. That is why most symptoms of the scoliosis describe symptoms of the fallen tarsal joint, such as one hip being higher than the other, back pain, fatigue, tilted shoulder line, one shoulder blade more prominent than the other, head sitting off centered, etc.

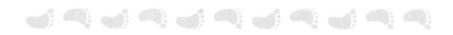

Bowlegs

When the tarsal joins fall laterally (supinate), the legs tend to tilt laterally also. This eventually can develop into the bowlegs. People with tight ligaments tend to develop this bowleg deformity.

Treatment: With the correct orthotics walk with the body weight on the medial arch by pulling the knees together. Walking with both feet at least shoulder width apart can straighten the knees while makes the body weight to fall on the medial arch. Also, massaging the medial side of the knees loosens up the tightened ligaments there, so can help to straighten the knees. Also, while sleeping using the 'bowlegs correction belt' can help.

Some people think cowboys develop bowlegs due to riding horses, or some Asian people think due to their parents piggybacked them around when they were kids. Then why do people who never ride horses or Americans or Europeans whose parents didn't piggyback them around develop the bowlegs? It is all due to the tarsal joint falling laterally and making the knees to go out.

Knock knees

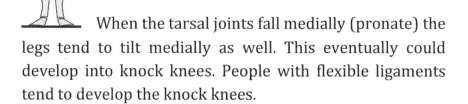

When the tarsal joints fall medially (pronate) the legs tend to tilt medially as well. This eventually could develop into knock knees. People with flexible ligaments tend to develop the knock knees.

Treatment: With the correct orthotics, try to walk with both feet together to straighten both knees. And while sleeping, holding a pillow between the knees with both feet together can help straighten the knees as well (or use the 'knock knee correction belt'). Also, massaging the lateral side of the knees can help loosen up the shortened ligaments and tendons to straighten the knees.

Our body is moldable with pressure or weight. The arch has been molded by our entire body weight all day against the flat floor. Now, we can mold the fallen arch back to its normal shape by pressing down over the correct orthotics with our entire body weight all day. Using the correct orthotics as early as possible can prevent all the above problems.

Also, all the brace treatments on the ankles, knees, or spine should be done with the correct orthotics. If not, bracing a joint can add more stress to the adjacent joints. Even toddlers who are born with any congenital problems should be fitted with the correct orthotics along with other treatments for the proper healing can take place with alignment from the feet up.

Chapter 13

Overall Body Performances

The fallen tarsal joint affects the overall body performance negatively. Let's go over some of the affected performances.

Limping

As mentioned earlier, both tarsal joints usually fall in different degrees and angles making one leg shorter than the other. With one leg shorter than the other, our body cannot avoid limping. Limping means moving our body without the alignment. This deteriorates the major weight-bearing joints while wasting lots of energy.

Treatment: The correct orthotics usually make the leg length the same by aligning both anklebones at the same height. Then our body can walk without limping. But for someone who has been limping awhile, it might take some time for the unbalanced muscles to adjust to the aligned joints.

Many people obviously limping do not know they are limping unless someone tells them so. Because that's how they have been walking since they were toddlers. Or some might admit they are limping but think that the reason for limping is the pain or discomfort in the back, knees, ankles, or in the foot. But, with the correct orthotics, the pain they thought causing the limping might disappear and they won't limp anymore.

In most cases, with the proper orthotics, both leg lengths become the same instantly and stretching the body in different directions as often as possible can speed up the muscle adjustment, then the leg muscles can develop with balance. With the same leg length, our body cannot limp, though we can pretend to be limping.

However, people with severe arthritis on the major weight-bearing joints, even with the correct orthotics, the leg length may not become exactly the same due to the damaged soft tissues between the joints and unbalanced rigid ligaments.

Yet, the leg length discrepancy will be noticeably reduced. Though, as long as they pass the AA test, their body functions with the physical balance. Also, people with cerebral palsy walk with much less swaying with the correct orthotics.

Falling

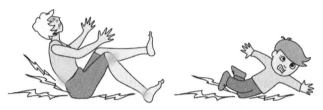

The more the fallen tarsal joint, the worse the body balance. This causes frequent falling. Most elderly people have severely fallen tarsal joints due to their tarsal joints being falling their entire lifetime, and kids' tarsal joint falls easily due to their still-growing-flexible foot ligaments. So, they tend to fall frequently.

Usually, slow-moving elderly people tend to fall backward on their hips and break the hip bones, and fast-moving kids tend to fall forward on their knees and get scratches on their skin. The hip bones are not just holding the muscular skeleton structure but also holding the entire internal organs like a shelf. Therefore, broken hips being pressed down with all those organs take more time to heal.

Treatment: The correct orthotics instantly provide the feet with balance. This significantly prevents the fallings.

Even with the correct orthotics, we can stumble over something and about to fall. But the correct orthotics give our body better chance to recover the balance before the fall.

Also, even though our body already fell, the body with alignment gets less damage than the body fell without the alignment. Another benefit is, with the correct orthotics, the healing will take place with alignment. Without the correct orthotics, the healing will take place without the alignment.

Some people doubt how the orthotics instantly provide the feet with balance and, thus, balance the entire body structure. This is like doubting how just putting the correct amount of air into the differently inflated tires instantly balance the tires and, thus, align the entire automobile.

Difficulty Standing Up from a Chair

As we get older the tarsal joint becomes more unstable as they keep falling. This will eventually make our body hard to stand up from a chair. The reason is, in order to stand up from a chair, we have to bend our body forward. This puts our entire body weight right onto the tarsal joint. This makes the tarsal joint to fall more tilting the anklebones worse. Then the body becomes more out of alignment. Then harder to muster up the strength. This makes standing from a chair difficult.

Treatment: The correct orthotics realign the fallen tarsal joints instantly aligning the anklebones at the same height and keep the tarsal joint from falling. This makes the body to utilize its full strength, so the body can stand up from a chair instantly much easier.

Difficulty Walking Uphill & Downhill.

Elderly people may have a hard time walking uphills or downhills due to the severely fallen tarsal joints.

Without the Correct Orthotics

When walking an uphill the body weight falls more on the heel side. And we need pull our body up through the fallen tarsal joint. But severely fallen tarsal joint makes it hard to muster up the strength to pull the body uphill. This makes it hard to walk the uphill.

When walking a downhill, the body weight pushes down at the front part of the anklebone on the sloping down ground. This makes the tarsal joint to fall more worsening the foot balance. So, the elderly body becomes more vulnerable to fall while walking downhills.

With the Correct Orthotics

With the correct orthotics, the tarsal joints are aligned and cannot fall on any terrain. So, the body can movie with alignment even walking the uphill. This allows the body to must up the full strength. So, walking the uphill becomes easier.

Even walking the downhill, with the correct orthotics, the tarsal joint cannot fall. So, makes it easy to walk down with confidence without worrying about falling.

Treatment: The correct orthotics keep the tarsal joints in alignment on any terrain. This makes our body to walk on any terrain with confidence and comfort.

Fatigue

On the fallen tarsal joints, our body moves without the alignment and constantly compensates until we lay down. This constant compensating waste quite a bit of our body energy, so our body tends to feel easily tired and can lead to the chronic fatigue.

Some people take energy-boosting substances without knowing that the energy from the substances make them do more activities with their misaligned body. This makes their major joints get more damage while the energy is leaking out all day through the misaligned joints. It's like, without the correct orthotics, everything is working against each other.

Treatment: The correct orthotics align the entire body structure from the feet up. This eliminates the zigzag standing, then the body doesn't have to compensate secondarily either. This saves the energy that was wasted for compensating primarily (zigzag standing) and secondarily (using the belly muscles, body-tilting, & toe-grabbing) all day long, so, our body becomes more energetic.

Muscle Weakness

There are two main ways to weaken the body muscles: not using them at all or keep using them without the alignment. But who doesn't use their muscles at all . . ? Unless for someone who's bedridden . . .

Without the correct orthotics the entire body muscles keep moving without the alignment. This affects the entire soft tissues negatively pulling and twisting around the misaligned joints. The soft tissues include the ligaments, tendons, muscles, nerves and blood vessels that run through the muscles, fascia that wrap around all the muscles and organs. Even though it is a slight twist, keep moving with this condition can negatively affect and eventually weaken the soft tissues.

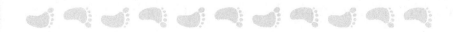

Also, when moving the body without the alignment, the nerves, the most delicate matter in our body, can be pulled or pinched between the misaligned joints and can get weakened and damaged by it. Once the nerves become weak, the body muscles become weak as well, since the nerves deliver the energy from the brain (the power generator of our body machine) to the muscles. So, when the nerves are damaged, even the massive muscles cannot move a thing. Also, the body moving without the alignment stresses the brain cells by constantly compensating in response to the signals from the peripheral nerves around the fallen tossal joint and around the misaligned joint due to the fallen tarsal joint.

Without the correct orthotics, the body with skinny and flexible muscles can go out of alignment much more than the body with thick and tight muscles. Also, people who cannot sit still and always move around doing something without the alignment can damage the tarsal joint more than sedentary people. This gives more chance for their muscles to become weak or atrophic down the road.

People with chronic pain, fibromyalgia, multiple sclerosis, lupus, Parkinson's disease, or stroke stricken are all having brain cells or the nerve problems. So, I suspect if the fallen tarsal joints might have something to do with those problems. It would be an interesting subject to research about. So, people with those problems might appreciate the correct orthotics more than any other people.

Chapter 14

Self-Checking

In This Chapter
- Which Tarsal Joint is Worse
- Hip Alignment Test
- Chain Reaction

How about getting to know our long-neglected tarsal joint . . . or the arch? There are a few ways to self-check our own tarsal joint. It just needs a close observation and palpation. As mentioned earlier, usually one tarsal joint falls more than the other, and discomfort or pain would mostly likely start with the side of the body with more-fallen-tarsal joint.

However, a few percentages of people start to have discomfort or pain in the foot with less- fallen-tarsal joint as the body compensates in a way to put more weight on the foot with less-fallen-tarsal joint before the pain starts with the foot with more-fallen-tarsal-joint. Let's find out which tarsal joint has fallen more.

Which Tarsal Joint is Worse

There are many ways to tell which foot has more-fallen-tarsal joint.

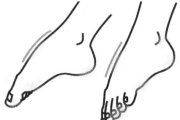

1, Look carefully and see which foot is slightly wider than the other foot. The wider foot most likely has more-fallen-tarsal joint.

2, If there are any foot deformities, such as bunion, hammertoes, curled toes, flat foot, etc., compare both feet and see which one is worse. The foot with worse deformity has more-fallen-tarsal joint.

3, While sitting down, extend (plantar flex) both ankles as much as possible. And observe the curved lines on top of both arches and see which one is flatter or less curved. The flatter or less curved arch has more-fallen-tarsal joint (the more curved arch has fallen as well just less than the other arch).

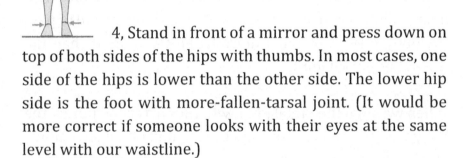

4, Stand in front of a mirror and press down on top of both sides of the hips with thumbs. In most cases, one side of the hips is lower than the other side. The lower hip side is the foot with more-fallen-tarsal joint. (It would be more correct if someone looks with their eyes at the same level with our waistline.)

5, The foot with more-fallen-tarsal joint also has a lower kneecap. So, while bending down at the waist, use index fingers and press up against under both kneecaps and see which one is lower. Also, if you have keen eyes, you might even be able to see which malleolus is lower by putting the thumbs on top of the medial malleoli, though the difference would be very minimal.

6, While walking, listen to the sound of each foot when it strikes the ground. We might hear one foot makes louder sound than the other the foot. The foot making louder sound is most likely with more-fallen-tarsal joint. The fallen tarsal joint weakens the ligaments and muscles of the foot, so, they cannot hold the foot bones tightly together. The foot with loosely connected bones makes louder sound when it strikes the ground.

7, When we are walking, usually one foot stays on the ground (the foot in the stance phase of the walking cycle) slight second longer than the other foot, which is the slight limping. The foot stays longer on the ground is the foot with more-fallen-tarsal joint. Because it takes longer time to pass the body weight through more-fallen-tarsal joint than the less-fallen-tarsal joint.

When we align the tarsal joint with the correct orthotics, the body weight can pass through the aligned tarsal joint much faster and easier. So, the walking and running can be faster and easier also.

8, Do the one foot at a time AA test without the orthotics and see how much weight each foot can lift before falling. The foot lifting less weight before falling has more-fallen-tarsal joint.

9, Measure the circumference of both legs or thighs with a measuring tape and see which one is thicker. Most likely the thicker side leg or thigh has more-fallen- tarsal joint. When the structure goes out of alignment, it gets shorter and thicker.

10, Observe the bottom of the foot and see which side foot has the toes closer to the ball of the foot. Most likely, the foot with the toes closer to the ball of the foot has more-fallen-tarsal joint.

11, Stand on the correct orthotics, and feel the pressure at the arch area of both feet. The foot with more support or pressure at the arch area has more-fallen-tarsal joint.

12, Make footprints of both feet and observe the width and length of the prints. Most likely the foot with longer and/or wider footprint and with more print at the arch area has more-fallen-tarsal joint.

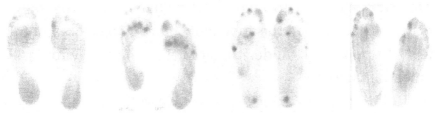

The above footprints are made with the Harris Mat foot imprinter. With these footprints, we can analyze how the body weight affects the bottom of the foot. Such as the flattening of the fatty tissues under the heel and the ball of the foot areas, how the metatarsal heads gone out of alignment, how the toes are grabbing the ground, and the indication of the bunion development, etc., which cannot tell just by looking at the foot from the outside.

Many people get confused when it comes to the alignment of our body, thinking that one leg shorter than the other is normal, the scoliosis causes the tilted hip bones, the spine is the one that controls the alignment of our entire body structure, and the height of the orthotics should be different for each foot since both feet look different or both tarsal joints fell differently.

Orthotics
Height

The height of the orthotics should be the same for both feet to align both anklebones at the same height. That is why the foot with more-fallen-tarsal joint feels more support under the arch than the foot with less-fallen-tarsal joint.

Hip Alignment Test

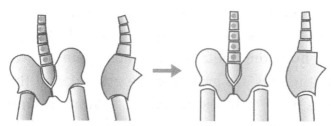

Most cases the correct orthotics systematically realigns the hip bones as well. This means the top of the sacrum on which the spine stands is aligned. After passing the AA test, the Hip

Alignment test (or HA test) can be done to see if the orthotics are aligning the hip bones as well.

The concept of the Hip Alignment test is the same as the AA test: applying weight on the hip bones.

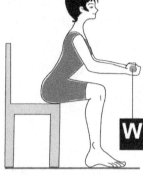 To do the Hip Alignment test, sit on the front edge of the chair and bring the shoulders forward to place both hands slightly in front of the feet (this makes the lifting harder, so makes it easy to check the back muscles strength) and slowly lift the weight without using the belly muscles.

On the tilted hip bones, the spine stands without alignment, so the entire back muscles cannot utilize the full strength, so makes it hard to lift the weight. On the aligned hips, the spine stands with alignment. This makes the entire back muscles can utilize the full strength in any angle within the range of motion, so makes the lifting easier.

However, if the back muscles are either very strong or very weak, we may not feel the dramatic difference with and without the correct orthotics. However, with the correct orthotics, we can feel less stress on the back joint.

Some people ask how the orthotics down under the feet can change the hip position while sitting on a chair. The hip bone is connected to all the way down to the anklebone even in a sitting posture. So, when the anklebone changes its angle, the leg bone changes its angle, then the thigh bone, then the hip bones. That is how the hip can be aligned starting from the anklebone with the correct orthotics under the feet.

Chain Reaction

Most people are perplexed when experiencing the strength with their own body with the correct orthotics, and some say, "How can the orthotics under my feet align my hips?" "Wow, my face angle really changed .. !!" "Oh, I can feel the weight gets lighter .. !!" And after people went home with orthotics reported me saying, "I wasn't able to walk even 15 minutes, and now with orthotics I can walk more than an hour without any problem." "My back (or knees) doesn't bother me anymore . . ." As if it's a miracle. But it's all a simply benefits of the alignment that works as a chain reaction that starts from the feet.

When I was preaching the importance of using the correct orthotics, someone who heard me enough said with a disapproving voice, "Then do you mean even people with cancer needs the orthotics?" I was speechless . . . it's like asking a car with an engine problem or transmission problem would need the tire alignment. Actually, those people need more energy than anybody to fight the disease, and we know the correct orthotics can give them a lot more physical strength too.

And did I mention another story of someone I know very well? She knows I am working with feet aligning people's anklebones, but not approve what I am doing, said one day her knees start hurting. So, out of pity, I told her she needs to align her both anklebones. And she told me as if I am dead wrong, "Inna, I said my knees hurt, not my ankles..!!" I was utterly stupefied . . !!!

Another story . . . but decent one. When I was fitting a young man of late 20s with the orthotics, I told him to step on the orthotics to do the AA test. And he stepped on the orthotics, and few seconds later he stepped down and stepped back on and stepped down all the while looking at the ceiling. And I looked at him and said, "What are you doing . . ?" and he said, "It's . . . freaky . . ." So, I asked frowning, "What do you mean . . ?" Thinking if there was a ghost. And he said, "When I stepped on, my knee pain disappears, and when I stepped down, my knee pain comes back . . ." A few minutes ago, I showed him the foot bone model with a leg bone stands on it. Couldn't he use different words, something like "Fantastic," "Amazing," or "Unbelievable," at least, but not "Freaky . . ?"

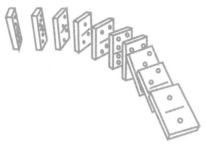

All of these are the simple chain reaction of the alignment, or the domino effect. When the tilted foundation is aligned, the entire structure aligns and becomes stronger and its range of motions becomes wider, and the structure functions better with less chance of injury than with the tilted foundation.

On the Internet, hundreds of X-ray images of ankle joints, knee joints, hips, and spines can be observed—most of them are not in alignment even after the joint replacement surgeries. The joints moving without the alignment is a serious problem. Though, no one raises any question . . . even healthcare professionals. Some might care about the alignment of our body but never talk about the "tarsal joint," or the "fallen tarsal joint," the very cause of all the above structural and mechanical problems.

Rather, many resources explain the symptoms of the fallen tarsal joint with the mechanical consequences of the fallen tarsal joint without mentioning the "fallen tarsal joint." It sounds kind of confusing, doesn't it . . ? Here is the example, "The back pain is from the pelvic rotation that causes the lengthening and shortening of the tendons or ligaments of the back." But the "pelvic rotation," is one of the alignment problems that is caused by the fallen tarsal joint. But no mention of the "fallen tarsal joint."

Furthermore, they explain the consequences of the fallen tarsal joint totally in an opposite way saying, "the pelvic obliquity has negative effects on the hip joint, knees, and feet, and even on the discs (excerpt from altlantotec.com/stilting of the pelvis section)." And another says, "Structural or functional problems in the legs, hips, or spine can cause a tilted pelvis. The most common causes are uneven leg lengths, spinal scoliosis, and muscle imbalance or contracture (healthgrades.com)." These are all consequences of the "fallen tarsal joint." But . . .

N0 ONE TALK ABOUT THE "TARSAL JOINT . . !!"

It seems the "Tarsal Joint" is a secret or a taboo . . .

There is a saying, *The truth is simple, but when you try to explain, it gets complicated.* That is what I did. So far, I spent so many words about the simple truth about the alignment: "The foundation goes out of alignment, the entire structure goes out of alignment."

Learning how to do the Anklebone Alignment test and finding correct orthotics, and shoes, and learn to walk correctly may sound complicated. But it's all about the alignment, a simple law of physics. Also, "The correct way is the simplest way." It'll be much simpler than keep taking painkillers or going through surgeries and still moving our body without alignment. Just eliminating the cause can get us back to the normal life right away.

I remember a 16-year-old student with autism who didn't talk much. While doing the AA test after fitting him with the orthotics, I asked him, "How do you feel?" And he was silent a while and I waited watching his expressionless face, and wondered if he was going to say anything. About 5 seconds later (which felt like 5 minutes) his answer started slowly with, "It's . . . like . . ." and he paused 3-4 seconds, and "Unlocking . . ." and another 3-4 seconds followed by, "The inner strength . . ." After I put his scattered words together, I was stunned by his insightful and accurate description of the event that just took place inside of his body. His major joints adjusting from their zigzag position to a straight position unlocked the strength that was trapped in the previous zigzag position . . !!

Also, it's kind of awe to hear some people say right after standing on the correct orthotics even before the AA test, "Oh, I am balanced . . !" or "Oh, my feet are balanced just now . . !" or "Wow, I just felt all my joints adjusting from the feet, my knees, hips . . . I felt they snapped back into alignment . . !!" I was amazed by those people who have the faculty to feel instantly their feet are balanced, or their body joints adjusting into alignment from the feet up, even though they have never experienced it before. Amazing body machine . . !!

Chapter 15

Body Machine's Agenda

Three Elements for Machine

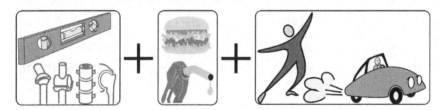

Every machine needs three elements to function properly: Alignment, Source of Energy (fuel or food), and Movement. All these three elements should be properly provided for a machine to function properly at its best. This also applies to our body machine. Let's go through more in detail with this common concept.

We don't want to put junk or wrong fuel into our car because it can sputter and stop running. For human body fuel, there are healthy food, junk food, and wrong or poisonous food. If we consume junk food, our body can get sick, and wrong or poisonous food can even end our life. Yes, good fuel is the one for every machine especially for our body health. So, we hear people are constantly talking about it—what to eat and how to eat.

How about the movement? If not moving, machines' joints become stiff and hard to move. Nowadays, due to machines taking over much of our physical work, people look for ways to move or exercise our body to maintain our body healthy, and there are countless places to go for all sorts of exercise.

Now, how about the alignment? We all know that the alignment is critical for any machine's performance and its lifespan. Therefore, all the man-made machines come out with alignment, and time to time, we check the alignment of those, especially expensive running ones, to avoid the risk of fixing the damages caused by driving them without the alignment.

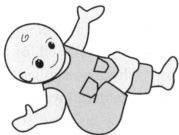

However, unlike man-made machines, the human body machine doesn't come out in a standing posture that needs the alignment, but, rather in a crumpled position. And it moves on its back or belly for about a year. During that time, the alignment is not necessary since the joints are not carrying the body weight. But...

When time comes and babes start venturing out to stand and walk, the tarsal joints collapse completely to the floor and become flat feet as shown in the photo here. Because toddlers foot bones are mostly cartilages with super-flexible ligaments. From the photo above, this kid's toes grabbing the ground is another sign of the fallen tarsal joint.

Small cookie-shape orthotics can prevent the toddlers' tarsal joints from falling and allow kids' foot bones to grow with the alignment alongside their entire body structure.

But people don't support kids' arches or the tarsal joint . . !! So, the human body has been growing, living, and dying without the alignment.

Another remarkable thing is that the pains that are caused by tilted anklebones or fallen tarsal joints, which are mechanical issues, are being treated mostly with chemicals—painkillers (actually they are "nerve-killers") or replacing the joints with man-made hardware (screws and plates), still without aligning the anklebones. So, our body deteriorates both mechanically and chemically at the same time—which makes the damage very complicated.

This makes the fixing of the problems very complicated without any chance to be done properly while the cost keeps piling up.

No wonder there are so many maintenance places—the hospitals—tried to fix the above structural and mechanical problems of the human body. If our body move with alignment with the correct orthotics, our society do not need this many human body maintenance places for all the above problems that are caused by the fallen tarsal joint.

Normal Damage & Extra Damage

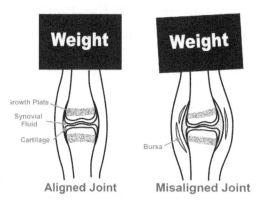

Even aligned joints deteriorate by weight all day. Let's call this deterioration the "normal damage." Thankfully, our body machine is to lie down at night for about 8 hours sleep. This gives every joint 8 hours of rest from 16 hours of weight-bearing task. Then the blood, the healing agent, can easily reach into the relaxed joints (open chain) delivering good things in and bad things out with each breath and heals the normal damage. So, technically, all the normal damage should mostly be healed while sleeping at night. As a result, the next morning, the body should be all refreshed and ready to function fully again.

But moving without the alignment definitely causes the "extra damage" on top of the "normal damage" in every weight-bearing joint and stresses all the ligaments around the misaligned joints as well. Then the 8 hours of sleep would not be enough to heal both the normal and extra damages, even though the healing agent works harder all night. This leaves our body to move next day with some residual damage that haven't been healed during the night's rest. And some people start to lay down more often than used to. Yet, most of us are not aware of this residual damage until it accumulated and becomes more than our body can tolerate; then pain suddenly starts. That is why we hear people say pain "suddenly" happened without any accident.

We can eliminate this "extra damage" by using the correct orthotics that align both anklebones at the same height.

Pregnant Women & Soldiers

Let's talk about how the fallen tarsal joint can affect the pregnant women and soldiers.

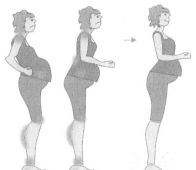

During the pregnancy, the tarsal joints fall much more severely than before the pregnancy due to the increasing weight and the pregnancy hormone, the Relaxin, loosens and relaxes most soft tissues of mom-to-be. This makes the body of mom-to-be more out of alignment causing the joint pain. This also can stress the babies in the womb, since babies feel all the stresses moms' experience, physically and emotionally. The correct orthotics can eliminate the stress from both making the pregnancy enjoyable.

Soldiers constantly walk, run, or jump during the training to prepare for battles. This causes their tarsal joins to fall more severely than most civilians. With the severely fallen tarsal joint, they go into battlefields carrying heavy equipment, plus occasionally, an injured comrade's body. While all the other equipment is aligned, the soldiers' body machines that handle the equipment are not aligned. So, they cannot utilize their full strength and move with the limited range of motions in their actions.

With the correct orthotics, soldiers' body can function with full strength and full range of motion, so they can walk, run, and jump longer and easier, and all the tasks can be performed with more accuracy without compensating. This also may save their own life and someone else's in some dire situations. Shouldn't be the correct orthotics the first equipment for soldiers' body alignment?

Two Legs to Three Legs to Four Legs

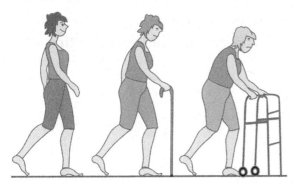

As we get older, the anklebones tilts more and more as the tarsal joints keep falling. This makes every weight-bearing joint out of alignment worse and worse making our body weaker and weaker. And at one point, our two feet are not able to carry our own body weight. Then we need extra foot and leg for help. So, we give up one hand to a cane, later, both hands on a walker, and might end up with our entire body on a wheelchair.

The correct orthotics can prevent or restore these problems. So, our own feet can carry our own body with confidence and comfort without those crutches as long as we live. For how long . . ? The "Instruction" from the human body Manufacturer says (in Genesis 6:3) 120 years long . . . though, some people might not like it . . . but with the correct orthotics, it might not be too bad . . .

As I mentioned earlier the orthotics are NOT crutches; they are the NECESSARY device for our body alignment to function properly without the crutches.

Body Vs. House & Automobile

With all the previous analyses, let's compare the problems of the fallen tarsal joints to the problems of a house on a tilted foundation, and an automobile with differently deflated tires.

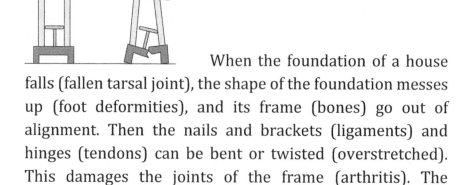 When the foundation of a house falls (fallen tarsal joint), the shape of the foundation messes up (foot deformities), and its frame (bones) go out of alignment. Then the nails and brackets (ligaments) and hinges (tendons) can be bent or twisted (overstretched). This damages the joints of the frame (arthritis). The

furniture in the house (organs) tilt to the one side (connective tissue stresses), the water pipes (blood vessels) and the electric wires (nerves) are pulled (stretched) to one sided, hang loose (contracted) on the other side. And the walls (skin) crack and sack (wrinkles) and the height of the house (body height) decreases. Then handymen (doctors) are very busy but oblivious to the fallen foundation (fallen tarsal joint). So, they won't be able to fix anything properly. So, fixing the same thing over and over (repeated treatment) without successes. In order to repair the house properly, the fallen foundation (fallen tarsal joint) must be fixed first with alignment (align both anklebones at the same height) by the foundation specialist (pedorthist) first.

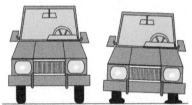 Now, an automobile with differently deflated tires (fallen tarsal joint) deforms the shape of the tires (foot deformity), and the automobile (our body) runs with the tilted body (limping). Then the joints of the automobile (body joins) damage (arthritis) much faster than their expected lifespan. Also, the belts and screws (ligaments) get twisted and pulled into wrong directions (overstretched) causing tension and stress. And driving the automobile without proper alignment uses more gas (waste of energy) as well. This will make the automobile (our body) to frequent the repair shops (hospitals) making the mechanics (medical staffs) super busy. And, eventually, end

up in a garage (in bed) or in a junkyard (in grave) much earlier than its manufacturer's designed lifespan. In order to fix the automobile in proper manner, those flat tires (fallen tarsal joint) have to be filled with right amount of air (correct orthotics aligning both anklebones at the same height) first to align the tires (tarsal joints).

When we spot an automobile running with tilted body, we hunk at the driver to let him know the tires need air. But when we see people limping, we just think that's the way they walk oblivious about the fallen tarsal joint. If we knew, wonder, would we tell them to get the correct orthotics?

Power of Aligned Anklebones

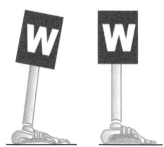 With the correct orthotics, we can test the power of the aligned anklebones with different exercise machines.

When lifting a weight, lift without the orthotics and with orthotics. And feel the different strength. With the correct orthotics, we can lift the same weight without using the belly muscles much easier and farther away from our body.

Work with a leg press machine without and with the orthotics. With the orthotics, our knee joints move much smoother with more power.

We can lift a weight with the legs, backs, or arms, and pushing and pulling in any postures (standing, sitting, or squatting down) without and with the orthotics and feel how our body become stronger with the orthotics.

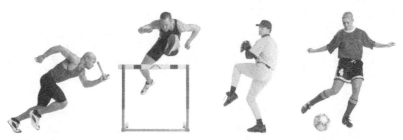

The human body is truly an amazing machine; truly fearful and wonderful . . . the most valuable asset of our lives. Look at all those athletes performing all kinds of activities: running, jumping, lifting, throwing, kicking, shooting, acrobatics activities . . . you name it. We even see 3 or 4 year old kids performing ice skating, and other activities that require extreme sense over the balance. Another amazing thing is that all those activities are being performed on the tilted anklebones—without the alignment or without the true physical balance. How much better our performances would be with the aligned anklebones, or with true physical balance . . ! Our body surely will produce much better work performance with less chance of injuries.

Hope many people become a pedorthist and soon understand the foot structure with weight bearing function and dispense the orthotics with "Anklebone Alignment Test," and busy aligning people's anklebones at the pedorthic offices at every corner of the streets with slogans saying, "Align both Anklebones at the Same Height," "Learn to Walk Correctly," or "Anklebone Alignment Test for Your Feet."

Wonder . . .

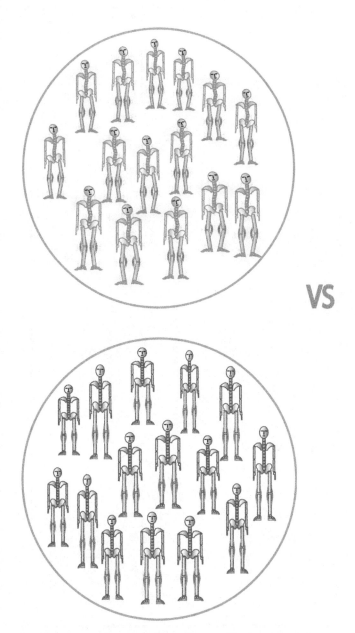

What will happen to the world when all the people on the earth are living with aligned body . . .

184

This diagram can help us to understand why most joint/muscle aches are related to not using the correct orthotics that align both anklebones at the same height.

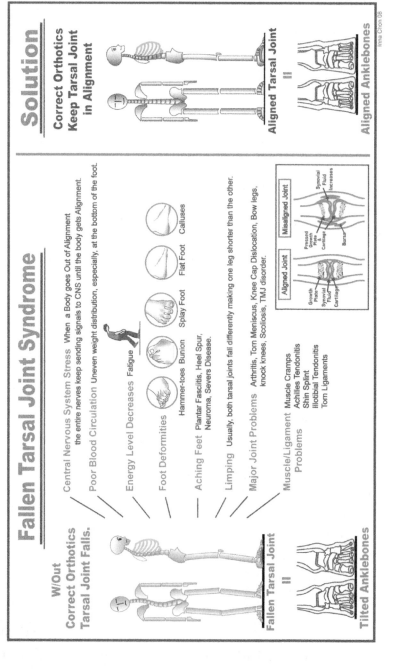

Fallen Tarsal Joint Syndrome

W/Out Correct Orthotics Tarsal Joint Falls.

Central Nervous System Stress When a Body goes Out of Alignment the entire nerves keep sending signals to CNS until the body gets Alignment.

Poor Blood Circulation Uneven weight distribution, especially, at the bottom of the foot.

Energy Level Decreases Fatigue

Foot Deformities
Hammer-toes Bunion Splay Foot Flat Foot Calluses

Aching Feet Plantar Fasciitis, Heel Spur, Neuroma, Severs Disease.

Limping Usually, both tarsal joints fall differently making one leg shorter than the other.

Major Joint Problems Arthritis, Torn Meniscus, Knee Cap Dislocation, Bow legs, knock knees, Scoliosis, TMJ disorder.

Muscle/Ligament Problems Muscle Cramps, Achilles Tendonitis, Shin Splint, Illiotibial Tendonitis, Torn Ligaments

Fallen Tarsal Joint =

Tilted Anklebones

Aligned Joint   Misaligned Joint

Growth Plate
Synovial Fluid
Cartilage

Pressed Growth Plate & Cartilage
Synovial Fluid Increases
Bursa

Solution

Correct Orthotics Keep Tarsal Joint in Alignment

Aligned Tarsal Joint =

Aligned Anklebones

Inna Chon 08

Epilogue

My research compelled by looking at the clustered side-by-side tarsal joints and its relation to the weight-bearing. Instantly, from an animator's viewpoint, I could analyze in my brain how our body weight transfers through the foot while walking. And I could see what is going to happen to the tarsal joint and its effect to the foot and the entire body structure. No wonder people are all limping, and I could imagine the damages the limping brings upon our body. And seeing the subtle compensating behaviors when we are lifting a weight came to the fruition in theorizing the compensating behaviors of our body due to the fallen tarsal joint and figuring out how to do the "Anklebone Alignment Test."

As people becoming more aware of the fallen tarsal joint, its debilitating effects on the foot and our overall health, and when the "Anklebone Alignment Test" finds its way to our daily life practice and healthcare practices, I believe the paradigm of our healthcare protocol would change. Because, when you think about, treating our body without aligning both anklebones at the same height doesn't make sense at all (it's like fixing a house on the unstable foundation).

There are much more to be explored in this pedorthic field; for example, advanced devices that can fabricate the orthotics while performing the Anklebone Alignment test, devices for the correct walking training, and brilliant ideas of orthotic holders for barefooted activities: such as gymnastic athletes, modern dancers, yoga practitioners, etc.

Also, clear orthotics materials with resilience to handle our body weight for fashionistas. Or, how about coming up with innovative orthotic materials that might resemble walking on the soft soil as in the Garden of Eden before the curse…?

Also, many schools should offer pedorthic courses with an enhanced curriculum incorporating the thorough analysis of the foot anatomy with the tarsal joint, how the body weight is related to the tarsal joint, and how to do the Anklebone Alignment Test. And many pedorthists should get busy aligning people's anklebones at every corner of streets. Now, not many schools offer pedorthic programs and the number of pedorthists are around 3 thousand in the U.S.A.—still dispensing orthotics without the Anklebone Alignment Test. Comparing to 30,000 plus optometrists in the U.S.A., the number of pedorthist should increase in a speedy way, because not everybody needs eyeglasses for the good vision since some people have the good vision without the eyeglasses, but everybody, including toddlers, needs orthotics if they like to move their body with alignment.

Most people still do not know or not clear about the pedorthic practice. I believe if the Anklebone Alignment Test is performed correctly by pedorthists when dispensing the orthotics and checking the shoe bottoms and teach people how to walk correctly, we are doing our job purposefully as our title "Ped-Orthist" claims to be. Then people would know clearly what the pedorthic practice is all about and seek help. Then more people can move their body with alignment.

Also, shoe manufacturers should start producing level-bottomed shoes, and make the average insteps a little higher than now to accommodate the restored arch height with the orthotics and incorporate small Velcro pieces inside of the shoes on the heel areas to hold the orthotics in place. This may prompt people to ask, "What are these Velcros for?" And get an answer like; "Didn't you know they are for the orthotics to align both anklebones at the same height?" This can help spreading the use of the orthotics faster.

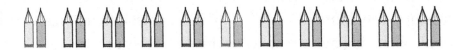

About the Author

"Inna" Chon is a Certified Pedorthist. She attended The Foot and Ankle Institute of Temple University, Philadelphia for her Pedorthic education. She majored in Physical Therapy in S. Korea where she grew up. Her work as an animator for Disney Feature Animation Studio for 16 movies developed skills to analyze movements with gravity and ground reaction forces the foot has to handle every day and the keen eyes to catch subtle movements. With these skills, she analyzes foot structure and its mechanics from a different point of view than the current medical study. Her analysis is based simply on the benefits of the alignment and disadvantages of the out of alignment.

While analyzing the foot structure with its functions of weight bearing and walking, she found out how to do the "Anklebone Alignment Test" and how to walk correctly. With this Anklebone Alignment Test and the correct walking, our body's physical balance can be restored and tested precisely, so, our body finally can move with alignment from the feet up, which is the true physical balance. This is a revolutionary discovery for our overall body health.

Educating people how to do the Anklebone Alignment Test and how to walk correctly is her passion in her quest to restore the human body's full mechanical functionality while bringing more respect to the pedorthic practice.

She now lives in Washington State where she enjoys many tall trees, islands, and umbrellas and rain boots—with the orthotics, of course.

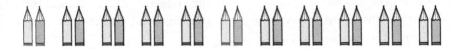

Index

Reference

Albert Einstein's Quote:
Retrieved from http://www.quote.net/quote/49509

Definition of Pedorthics and Pedorthist:
Retrieved from
http://www.oandpcare.org/PedorthicCareFaq

Orthotics can Help Kids' Growing Pains (2012):
Retrieved from
http://www.pedorthic.ca/orthotics-can-help-kids-growing-pains

The Fascinating History of the Orthotics (2006):
Retrieved from
http://www.biotechpossibilities.com/fascinating-history-foot-orthotics

The cause of tilted hip being shortening of the hip flexor
and lengthening of the hip extensor, or changing shape
of the spine (2017):
Retrieved from http://www.medicalnewstoday.com

Excerpt "pelvic obliquity has negative effects on hip
joints, knees, and feet, and even the discs." (2017):
Retrieved from altlantotec.com/tilt

Acknowledgements

I am so grateful to come to the point of writing this end part of the book. I know it's the "Manufacturer of the foot" who started me on this task; He showed me the things I needed to see for this task from the start and sparked a passion in me that energized me through it all. So, I say, "Thank You, the Master of the Engineer," for entrusting me in this task and help me through the occasional dispiriting moments.

Secondly, I send my gratitude to my husband who introduced the pedorthic field to me without foreseeing that his wife would soon fall in love with the foot and had to listen to her talking about the foot, "ALL THE TIME."

Lastly, I like to acknowledge many kind people who willingly listened to my ongoing talk about the foot, and another many kind people who blocked their ears to my restless foot talk; so, I could rest for the next opportunity.

If any organization or a group like to hear me out what I get to say about the foot, contact me at:

innachon2@yahoo.com, or call/text @ 360. 762. 5227

"Inna" Chon, Pedorthist.

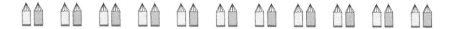

The Truth will Set You Free

Made in United States
Orlando, FL
21 August 2024

50614111R00114